Psoriasis: Free and Clear

Psoriasis: Free and Clear

USING FOOD AND POSITIVE ENERGY TO HEAL YOUR SKIN

*   *   *

Marjy Berkman

Dedication

I WANT TO GIVE THANKS to the major influences for this book, who have inspired me for years to wake up to a healthier life. They are my very supportive mom and dad, my sister Ellen, my niece Joey, Brigitte Mars, Michael Shulkin, Holly Edwards, Elisa Byler, Eckhart Tolle, Abraham and Esther and Jerry Hicks, Louise Hay, Matt Kahn, Lenny Christopher, Nick Good, Lyna Norberg, Byron Katie, Barbara Norberg, and Nassim Haramen.

Contents

Introduction

*"Truly, the greatest gift you have to give is
that of your own self-transformation."*

— LAO TZU

I AM WRITING TODAY BECAUSE I have to. This information must be shared. This life, this precious life, is in our hands, literally. We each have the ability to help create the life we want.

The challenges that come up for us, the difficulties and hardships, can show us what is going on within our bodies and turn out to be gifts that have a beautiful treasure for us. They can awaken our souls to our life's joys and our highest potential.

For me, my skin has always been my messenger, guiding me toward empowerment. From age nineteen to age forty-two, I had psoriasis on my body—thick, red patches that launched me on an epic health journey. Then the psoriasis disappeared.

Our very intelligent bodies are reflections of what is going on within us. We are incredible maps on which our emotions, ailments and challenges are shown as a guide to our inner world. They guide us into ourselves, giving us information and a reflection of that which is trying to get our attention. The same is true of our skin. Psoriasis showed me my inner hardships and helped me look at the shadows that had not been addressed or brought to awareness. These shadows were my hidden emotions and fears, and the part of me that was craving attention and love.

My journey to heal psoriasis was not an easy one. I struggled and resisted and did not want to face that this was my reality. I secluded myself from the world and did not want to change my ways. Then I started to see an opportunity for relief and healing. One step at a time, I experimented with different foods, supplements, lifestyle changes, and different practices to help me feel good, love myself, feel my emotions, and eventually tap into a larger part of myself—my spirit. I began to see that I was going to be okay, and—more so—that clear skin was possible.

Psoriasis: Free and Clear is not only about psoriasis and the steps you can take to help clear your skin but also about the massive potential that we have as humans to transform our lives. It is about how to thrive through excellent nutrition and connection to the spirit within. If you have psoriasis, this book can change your whole viewpoint of this disease and why it is in your life. It will offer you tangible tools and tips to help heal your body.

I wrote this book because I discovered that you could help create your reality based upon your beliefs and what you choose to focus on. By directing your energy and focus consistently and deliberately to positive feelings, peace, ease, and things that make you feel good, you begin to emanate a certain state that attracts more of the same. Bringing these feelings into your daily experience regularly is helpful in attracting more experiences that match those feelings. Then, you can more easily return to this state again because your body has a certain intelligence and remembrance of this experience. At the same time, we have emotions of anger, sadness, frustration, and fear. By not avoiding and resisting these emotions, by instead allowing them and loving yourself through them, you feel profound self-acceptance. This self-approval also creates a field of energy that is soft and loving, in which a deep healing can take place. Loving myself in the face of all of these emotions was—and still is—a practice and tool that I have developed and continue to develop each day. This practice can create great healing and can help you in clearing your skin.

I offer my story and twenty-three years of self-experimenting, research, lifestyle adaptations, and guidelines. My intention is to expedite your healing process, help you find peace with your situation, and offer you inspiration in your daily life. I did it, even though there were many times I didn't think I could.

I invite you to read this book with an open heart. Know that you were drawn here for a reason, and that I am offering you a perspective on skin challenges that can help you find peace where you are and maybe even heal your skin. I wish someone had told me back then, when I discovered that I had psoriasis that there was another way besides settling into having it for life. After healing myself, I am here to say that there is hope; there is a possibility for you to experience a breakthrough in your life. Your journey will be unique to you and—while I am not claiming a cure for psoriasis—I can share with you what worked for me.

The first chapter discusses the definition and causes of psoriasis.

CHAPTER 1

What is Psoriasis?

* * *

PSORIASIS IS A NON-CONTAGIOUS SKIN disease that affects about 4.5 million people in the US. It is characterized by red, dry plaques, or scaling, of skin that occur commonly on elbows, knees, and scalp and can occur elsewhere in the body, including on the palms of the hands, soles of the feet, and under the finger and toenails. Rarely, you can find psoriasis in skin folds, inside the mouth or on genitals. It usually shows up around injury sites as well and can range from mild to severe.

Psoriasis can show up in different ways for different people. It can be red or pink with areas of thickened, raised and dry skin; small flattened bumps; large thick plaques of raised skin; pink, mildly dry skin, or big flakes that fall off. There are several different types of psoriasis including psoriasis vulgarism or plaque psoriasis (the common type); guttate psoriasis (small, drop-like spots); inverse psoriasis (in the folds of the underarms, navel, and buttocks); pustular psoriasis (pus-filled yellowish, small blisters), and palmoplantar psoriasis (on the palms and soles).

The scales come from a rapid proliferation of skin cells that is triggered by abnormal lymphocytes in the blood. Cells replicate at a normal rate every twenty-eight to thirty-two days, but with psoriasis, cells replicate every three to four days, without the skin sloughing off. There can be cycles of flare-ups and remission.

CAUSES

HERE ARE SOME OF THE MANY POTENTIAL PHYSICAL CAUSES OF PSORIASIS:

- Improper detoxification and overwhelming toxicity in the body
- A genetic component
- Faulty fat metabolism
- Emotional trauma, which may be an initial trigger. Trauma can arise from difficult emotions such as shame and fear or from a situation that is hard and challenging.
- A streptococcal infection that has been recently active (2-3 weeks prior). This infection triggers guttate psoriasis specifically.

One thing that is known is that there is an immune component. Psoriasis is considered to be an autoimmune condition. This means the body's immune system attacks its own tissues. T-cells, produced by the body, attack the skin cells, causing swelling and reddening. This causes the body to try to heal itself by quickly producing, or over-producing, skin cells. This leads to scales and thickening of the skin. The immune system seems to mistake the skin for a pathogen.

SOME CAUSES OF AUTOIMMUNE DISORDERS ARE:

- Stress
- Chronic infection
- Allergies
- Poor nutrition
- Vitamin D deficiency

With autoimmune conditions such as psoriasis, it is necessary to regulate the immune system, which could be overactive, lower inflammation, and fight infection.

The digestive system is a huge part of this. Since much of the immune system is located in the gut, and digestion plays such a large role in the whole health of the body, healing the gut is crucial to healing psoriasis and any autoimmune disease.

THINGS THAT CAN AGGRAVATE PSORIASIS INCLUDE:

- Cold weather
- Stress
- Alcohol
- Smoking
- Hormone fluctuations
- Food allergens
- Bacterial or viral infection
- Dry air
- Some medicines, including beta-blockers and lithium
- Injury to the skin

Before we embark on the journey to clearing your skin by focusing on the physical, emotional, and spiritual components that need attention, I would like to share my story.

CHAPTER 2

My Journey

* * *

I WAS A VERY DIFFERENT person before I developed psoriasis. It seems like a life-time ago now. As a teenager, growing up in an affluent section of Pittsburgh, Pennsylvania, I was scared, confused, and hid from my emotions. I craved some sort of connection to something, anything. I always wanted to get high or escape reality. I started drinking alcohol in high school, at the age of fifteen. I had a large group of friends, and we liked to "party." I generally felt depressed and uncomfortable in my body and sought a way to find relief, and alcohol lifted me. I drank as an escape from reality because I did not know how to handle the fear, confusion, and depression I was feeling, nor did I know how to handle the general emotions of life. My parents did the best they could to support me, yet I still struggled.

I was insecure and lacked confidence: this stemmed from me not find-ing value in who I was. I didn't see that I had anything to offer except the fact that I was pretty. I compared myself to my sister, who was very intelligent. I, on the other hand, had average grades and lacked inter-est in school. I was also uninspired by what I was introduced to, such as the news on television and the discussions around me, often political in nature, and events that were going on in the world. Back then, I inter-preted my lack of interest as unintelligence because I had little to contrib-ute. This made me feel terribly uncomfortable, especially growing up in a home with very well-educated people.

I also happen to be a very sensitive person, and an empath, mean-ing I feel things deeply and can sometimes tap into what others are feeling. I had a difficult time handling the emotions that arose around being different, being so sensitive, and being uninspired by school and the normal societal expectations of youth. I had yet to discover that I had something to contribute, so I always felt insecure. I could not grasp that there might have been something that would ignite my passion for life.

As I look back, I imagine that I may have had a hormonal imbalance as well. I believe I was lacking some of the "feel-good" hormones, such as endorphins. I have never had this tested but considering my symptoms and depression, this could have been the case.

I was not turned on by life, was disengaged from my body, and felt very alone.

In 1989, I was nineteen years old, studying English Literature in my second year of college at the University of Wisconsin. I woke up one morning very itchy, and knew right away something was wrong. With shock and horror as I looked at my skin, I discovered thick red-silver scaly blotches covering my body. I was terrified. A lot of emotion came to the surface all at once. I felt fear and anger and was in a state of panic.

What could it be?

I immediately grabbed the phone to call my mom. "Mom, something has happened! I am covered in I don't know what!" I told her. I did have earlier symptoms of acne when I was a young teenager, but nothing like this. Psoriasis showed up literally overnight.

I flew home to my family in Pittsburgh to get checked out. My dad was a doctor who had a lot of connections so we went to a dermatologist right away. I recall sitting in his office waiting for the diagnosis with my mom, feeling terribly vulnerable and confused. The doctor came out and told me I had psoriasis and explained what it was. He proceeded to tell me something that has impacted my life dramatically. He told me I would have this disease for life, that it was incurable.

Feeling hopeless and devastated, it seemed then and there that I had entered a living nightmare and that my world had just fallen apart. "For life" and "incurable" reverberated in my body. Feelings of total despair arose in that moment as I heard the news that there was no cure for this disease covering my skin.

This is the kind of devastation you have when circumstances happen to you and you believe you have no control over your reality. It seemed there was nothing that I could do to change this and I just wanted out of my skin and to find some relief from the despair I felt.

A CHALLENGING TIME

The day I found out I had psoriasis and the doctor told me it was incurable forever changed the path of my life. I left the office a mess, my mom consoling me, telling me everything would be okay. My mom was, and is, always supportive and present no matter what the challenge. She was one of those moms who was born to be a mom, couldn't wait to be one, and loved and cared for her children with everything she had. But I couldn't hear that everything was going to be okay then. All I could hear was that this thing was happening to me; this skin disease was here for good. I felt as if my world had collapsed. All that I had known vanished in an instant.

I hit a deep depression filled with anger and frustration, which lasted for the next few years. I had been told my whole life that I was beautiful and I believed this to be my gift. Now I was covered in these spots and patches, I didn't look so pretty anymore. In addition to the psoriasis, I was physically very unhealthy. Before I developed psoriasis, I had asthma, acne, gastroenteritis, depression, and many hip surgeries early in my life. All of these diseases showed up at different times before I went to college. I was walking a slightly dangerous path, mindlessly living my life and numbing myself with drinking. I still didn't know how to feel emotions that were deep or uncomfortable.

THE NEXT PHASE

After my initial diagnosis, I spent the next five years, until 1994, adjusting to the appearance of my skin. I had a difficult time coming to terms with my psoriasis and wished it away constantly. Of all the health issues I'd had in my life, this one was the most challenging because it was so noticeable. After some time, the psoriasis mostly settled on my joint areas on my knees, elbows, and hips. It grew very thick in those areas, and it barely changed at all in the twenty-three-years I suffered with it.

I was a young woman very led by her ego and need for love and approval from others. With psoriasis now on my body, I thought I looked like a monster. I was totally focused on these patches, aware of their presence at all times, especially when they were exposed. I was embarrassed and ashamed and felt terribly ugly and deformed. I walked around feeling as if there was a spotlight on my skin . . . and on me. I judged myself harshly because I felt different from everyone else. This self-judgment only served to isolate me more while I deeply longed to feel "normal." I dreaded spring and summer since wearing short-sleeved shirts and shorts meant my skin would be exposed and people would see my red scaly patches. I tried to hide them by keeping my skin covered in the warm days of spring and summer, even when I was hot, uncomfortable, and sweating. I would wear long-sleeved shirts and long skirts or pants—basically anything to hide the psoriasis.

I believed that no one could possibly love me like this, that I was unlovable. The loneliness was terrifying. Then, I found some inspiration.

NEW HOPE

When the doctor first diagnosed me, he told me right away that cortisone would help take the discomfort away and also make the psoriasis much less noticeable. Relieved that there was an option to help make it look better, I started cortisone shots right away, and continued for multiple times. But what I discovered about the shots is that they only helped temporarily. The patches would subside, and then come back within a few days, sometimes worse than when they began. I also developed a scar on one of those patches that looks like an indention on my shin from the cortisone shot. It was clear that the cortisone was not reaching the core cause at all. I began to believe that my psoriasis would never go away if I just kept receiving shots, and worried what side effects they may have. In my heart, I knew there had to be another way.

Then one day, I was eating pizza for lunch, and I felt just awful. I was nauseous and noticed my skin had broken out with acne. It was hard for me to look at myself and not get upset. I felt depressed and anxious at the same time, wanting to scream. I began to wonder if there may be a link between what I was eating and the skin problems. I had known people with very healthy eating habits, who ate lots of organic veggies and fruit, and thought about how healthy and vibrant they looked. I began to wonder if some of my habits were being reflected through my skin. I realized that there may be a connection there, and I immediately felt some relief from my ongoing frustration. I asked myself, could it be that what I was putting in my body was wreaking havoc? This really was an epiphany for me because I had never before made that connection. It was as if a huge door opened up with bright, gold lights shining out from it and endless possibilities waiting on the other side. I opened that door up right then and decided to look for someone who had information on nutrition and health.

And so I began my research into holistic health.

I was 24 in 1994, living in Boulder, Colorado. Boulder is a Mecca for holistic studies, with many health teachers, schools, and practitioners of holistic medicine. I looked in the phone book and found someone who could help me with my nutrition and check to see if I had food allergies. She was a nutritionist and also offered acupuncture and Chinese herbs. Her name is Lyna Norberg, and I will never forget her; she helped steer me toward making more nourishing choices for my body. Lyna was very loving and nurturing, and I felt comfortable being vulnerable with her while telling her my story. She gave me acupuncture and then tested me for food allergies as well. She told me there were some lifestyle changes I could make that would really help me, including getting off wheat, dairy, and alcohol.

Well. Can you say resistance? Holy... No way! Her suggestion put me in a very defensive, reactive mode. I refused to accept these suggestions and left her office very angry and rude, saying, "Fuck, no." I was upset by just the thought of giving up those things that had been such a part of my life, even though I saw that I needed to make some changes. After that appointment with Lyna, I was angry at her suggestion but, deep down, I was more afraid that I would not be able to accomplish such a feat. I felt threatened. I also felt challenged because I was comfortable in the lifestyle I'd been in for so long and did not want to let it go.

But Lyna had planted a seed by offering me such valuable information. It was up to me to take the next steps and go back to her and experiment with her suggestions.

About a year after my first meeting with Lyna, I chose to let go of the foods she suggested I eliminate; first, I stopped eating gluten and dairy. Then, I eliminated soy, eggs, refined sugars, grains, and alcohol. I didn't eliminate these foods and lifestyle habits all at once; rather I let go of one or two at a time. I didn't let go of some foods until years later. I was someone who needed to take baby steps. Well, Lyna had been right; I started seeing changes in my health.

As I got off dairy, my asthma disappeared almost instantly. By getting off gluten and grains, the irritable bowel syndrome, which I developed during college, disappeared. When I let go of soy, alcohol, and refined sugars, the acne on my skin dramatically improved. After witnessing these results, I began to see that food and alcohol were causing havoc in my body.

Was it easy? No. It was especially hard in the beginning. But I went slowly, at a pace that worked for me. I would have given up or tried anything for the sake of healing myself. I chose to let go of things that were not helping me thrive. I started to see that what I ate and drank directly affected my health. Basically, my body was reacting to a lifetime of low nutrition and, at this point, malnutrition.

In 1995, soon after I'd been to see my nutritionist, I decided to dive into herbal studies and went back to school for herbalism in Boulder. My intention was to learn more about healing my self, and specifically psoriasis. I spent the next two and a half years in study, focusing on discovering ways to heal the body.

Over time, as I started to see results, I realized that there is always a way. There is always a path toward relief, toward ease, toward health. Even if you are in an acute situation and cannot see your way, there is a path; you may just not see it yet. The possibilities are endless in this vast universe, in any situation; just because we may not see them yet does not mean they don't exist.

After I made all these changes, I began to realize how powerful, strong, and determined I am. I also realized that if you are giving something up, such as wheat or alcohol, it really helps to find substitutes to take the place of these things. This could be new healthy drinks or bread-alternatives. I offer a list of healthy options in Chapter 4, Part 2 "Physical Healing." The art of decision-making really comes into play here. The journey to healing is all about paying close attention to the options laid out for you and then making decisions that will really nourish and satisfy your needs.

All of the success and healing I began experiencing as a result of my dietary changes felt rewarding. I continually experimented with different herbs and healing modalities as I was getting more comfortable in my body. I was inspired by learning in a school setting and later went on to become an esthetician, nutritionist, and raw chef. All these roles unlocked different keys to learning the alchemy that would help heal my skin. I also continually experimented with ways of eating that would continue to support me in this healing process. I started off doing a macrobiotic diet while I was studying herbs--eating a lot of rice, miso, tofu, and fish. Some friends and teachers I knew inspired me to stop eating meat and fish and go vegan. Then, after being strongly inspired by David Wolfe and many of his books, which I mention in my resource section, I went 100% raw for seven years. During this time, I also experimented with being a fruitarian, living mostly on fruit and some leafy greens. Then, when I lived on Kauai, Hawaii, I started eating a more Paleolithic-type diet of fish and meat. The psoriasis was still there, but I was determined to find a way to say goodbye to it.

I moved to Kauai with my partner when I was 38 years old, in 2008. We left our lives in Boulder to try out island living. My main reason for moving there was to see if psoriasis would heal in a warm, humid climate. Well, it didn't. In fact, I developed a skin condition in which I had weeping sores on my legs and face. It was terrifying. I was afraid I would have this condition forever and felt vulnerable in such a consistently warm climate, with my skin constantly exposed for others to see. This was one of the most difficult times for me. This led me onto a deep spiritual practice where I discovered the power of the spirit that is alive within us to heal.

I started meditation a few years before moving to Kauai and, while there, continued my practice. I could not believe how busy my thoughts were, as I sat watching what arose, and allowing everything. I began attempting to conjure emotions and feelings with the intention of raising my vibration. I started reading the book, *The Vortex* by Esther and Jerry Hicks. This was another pivotal time for me because I began to realize the essential benefit of feeling good and, also, where to direct my attention and focus. I realized that my energy field attracted like energy and that if I was feeling at peace consistently then peaceful situations followed. Soon the weeping sores went away, thankfully; that seemed to be connected with the new, increased calmness I was beginning to feel in my life.

I eventually moved back to Boulder, a completely different person. In 2012, I went to school again, and this time I studied massage. This was a profound time for me, as studying massage was about getting comfortable with being seen and touched. I gained tremendous confidence and comfort through practice in receiving massage and being witnessed with a skin disease. I went on to teach at the school, which was a great accomplishment. Before this time, I'd always said "No" to basically anything that meant I had to talk in front of people. Soon, I faced my lifelong fear of public speaking, teaching nutrition at this wonderful, eclectic school, The Berkana Institute of Massage Therapy.

At the same time, I was suddenly feeling what some call their "superpower" skills, their "super-heroine powers", so to speak. So instead of shrinking from the opportunity because of fear of disapproval and lack of confidence, I chose to go for it. I had previously been given quite a few opportunities to teach, and I had always shrunk from it. Now I was ready to allow my voice to express, to let my spirit shine, to trust that I had something to offer, even if it meant stumbling through it at first, turning bright red, or stuttering. This was a rite of passage for me as I stepped into my power. Once I faced my ultimate fear, I would know that I could do anything. Utilizing all of the skills I had developed through studying different inspirational teachers, I taught my first class in holistic studies. This was 2012; that same year, I noticed one day that my psoriasis was gone.

WHY I DEVELOPED PSORIASIS
THERE ARE MANY FACTORS THAT I BELIEVE LED TO THE MANIFESTATION OF PSORIASIS ON MY BODY.

* Up until the point where I began my journey to health, I did whatever I felt like, ate whatever I wanted, drank alcohol, and smoked cigarettes. I had a difficult time setting limits in my life. I just kept on partying and making choices that may have not been the best for my body.
* My immune system was overactive and began to attack itself, unable to handle the lifestyle I was living.
* I was undernourished.
* I was thinking a lot of negative thoughts, often about myself. I was feeling insecure, disempowered, and disconnected from my inner source much of the time.
* I was bulimic prior to developing psoriasis and was physically harming my intestines and body.
* I did not love myself.
* I had some relatives who also had skin problems; hence, there was a genetic component.
* I had recently gotten off cigarettes, coffee, and stopped being bulimic. This may have sent my body into a healing crisis.

* I was an anxious person a lot of the time, under constant stress with life and school.

Now that you know more about the underlying causes of psoriasis and my journey, we can begin to talk about the art of self-healing.

CHAPTER 3
The Art of Clearing Skin

∗ ∗ ∗

NOW THAT YOU KNOW A little bit more about me and the challenges I have faced having psoriasis, as well as the good that has found its way into my life because of it, let's start to dive into how this transformation happened for me.

Clearing your skin is truly an art. Some folks are artists who paint. Some are artists of words or clay or dance. I am an artist of transformation. Others may call me an alchemist. Whatever the name, I have found a way to live and be in this world that has allowed me to transform my health and my skin. I decided to look at psoriasis as an opportunity for discovery to learn about my body, my potential, and myself. As I did so, the psoriasis disappeared from my body, and I, therefore, have learned a true art: self-healing. I know that I have much more to learn and uncover in this life, yet I am fulfilled and enchanted by this amazing capability of our bodies and minds.

The following is what I learned about clearing skin.

Our difficulties and challenges in life can cause issues on our skin. Our bodies are direct mirrors of what is going on within us, physically and emotionally. They reflect what is within in multiple ways.

First of all, if there is a strong emotion stuck in the body because it has not been processed or truly felt, then it needs a place to go. If we are on overload with our feelings, in the habit of suppressing them, then the emotions get stored in our bodies and can end up erupting through the skin as acne, psoriasis, eczema, etc. We live in a society

14

that generates a tremendous amount of stimuli, and is filled with events and interactions, and the emotions that follow. This often leads to unprocessed feelings, which may result in a physical reaction. My particular body reacts through my skin. For other people, it could show up as another physical ailment. It could be arthritis, chronic back pain, or many other illnesses. My skin shows me clearly when I have unprocessed feelings.

Second, with psoriasis, you are experiencing an autoimmune condition and likely some other imbalances, which show up as rapid replication of skin. Your body is overproducing skin cells partially because its own imbalanced immune system is attacking the skin.

Third, when it comes to skin challenges like psoriasis, the imbalance is there for you to see. It reminds you continually to take a closer look, that something needs attention, that something in your body is in need of more love; whether physical, emotional, or spiritual, something is calling out for attention.

Having my challenge manifest right there on my skin for the world to see was the impetus for me to change my lifestyle as I did.

Through my journey I've come to see my psoriasis as a blessing. Initially, this may sound insane, yet once you shift your perception, you can see the benefit. What has shown up on your body is something that really needs attention, love, forgiveness and acceptance. Psoriasis may be a manifestation of our wounds, of our emotional traumas and challenges, showing us that we need to give this nourishing attention to our bodies. It is an invitation to deepen your love for yourself. You are the best person to offer this care, and the best medicine we can offer is tender love toward ourselves.

I will go into tools and tips to find true self-love and work on the emotional aspect of healing psoriasis in Chapter 5, Emotional Healing. I know it isn't easy, and this stage will take time, but I encourage you to see the blessing in the discomfort, the beauty in the patches, and the breakthrough in this skin disease. This can feel impossible, especially if you are in a flare-up, or have been dealing with skin issues for many years.

Yet, why not try taking a deep breath and creating a new pathway? To create a new pathway, start with being gentle with yourself as you gather your tool belt, so to speak, which includes practices and inspirations that help and inspire you. By being willing to do something different, by taking it one step at a time, by following your inspiration and having some go-to strategies to help you through a difficult time, you are already creating new patterns. You can pick one thing to play with at a time, and practice adding that into your life. I will go more deeply into tools and practices in my chapter on Empowerment Tools.

THE THREE ASPECTS OF HEALING PSORIASIS

The next three chapters cover three components of the steps I took to heal my psoriasis. I focused on three elements of healing; Physical Healing, Emotional Healing, and Spiritual Healing.

1. **Physical Healing:** I started out looking solely at what I could do on a physical level. The first thing I focused on, and continued for most of my journey, was how I could change my nutritional and lifestyle choices, as well as add in supplements and exercise. I will share with you what I learned and implemented in Chapter 4: Physical Healing.

2. **Emotional Healing:** Chapter 5: Emotional Healing addresses the impact that emotions have on psoriasis. In this chapter, I'll show you tools and practices to love and accept yourself and pay attention to your emotions. This may be a necessary step toward your personal peace and happiness in your life or the next move toward your dream, whatever that may be. It is often the key to shifting people's lives.

3. **Spiritual Healing:** In the chapter on spiritual healing, Chapter 6, I discuss lifestyle practices to create the life you want and find peace with or without psoriasis.

Unfortunately, it is not as easy as taking one pill to rid our bodies of psoriasis. There is usually not just one piece to the puzzle of healing our bodies. Each person will have his or her own group of things that come together and create healing.

So we will begin our discussion in the next chapter: Physical Healing.

CHAPTER 4

Physical Healing

*   *   *

LET'S BEGIN WITH THE PHYSICAL aspect of healing psoriasis, which includes the following sections:

1. Your Relationship with Food, Gut Health, and Digestion.
2. Nutritional Guidelines; lists of things to eat and drink and what to avoid, a list of superfoods, and food substitutes.
3. Using Supplements and Herbs in Healing.

For me, working in the physical realm was the most obvious place to begin because the psoriasis was on my body, on my physical being. As I said earlier, my body was reacting to a lifetime of low nutrition and, eventually, malnutrition. I began to realize that what I ate and drank directly affected my health. Once I began working with my nutritionist, I began to become more aware of what was going on day-to-day in my body. As I paid closer attention to the relationship between what I ingested and the possible reactions that followed, I felt excited and empowered by this knowledge.

This information may help you upgrade your body so that it is optimally fed and nourished to the point that disease cannot live in the healthy environment you have set up for yourself.

PART 1
YOUR RELATIONSHIP WITH FOOD, GUT HEALTH, AND DIGESTION

*"The health of a cell is a reflection of the
environment in which the cells live."*

—BRUCE LIPTON

Food. Oh how I love thee! Discovering the alchemy of foods that really support me in thriving has been my focus for more than two decades. I have tried just about every nutritional regimen there is. I have been macrobiotic, vegan, 100% raw, fruitarian, paleo, and now I have come to a place of knowing what works for me and helps me to look and feel amazing. Basically, it is a combination of all of these.

The single most important thing I want to pass on in regard to food is that there may be things you are ingesting and taking in that simply *do not work for you,* which is a great place to start on this journey of health and clearing your skin. What foods are not helping you to thrive? Discovering the answer to this very important question can help you toward the healing of your skin. Often you will see changes right away. Let's bring awareness first to your relationship to food.

DISCOVERING YOUR CURRENT RELATIONSHIP TO FOOD

Developing a healthy relationship to food and eating has been a large part of the journey for me. I was an anxious person growing up and I brought this with me to the dining table.

I have been a worrier for as long as I can remember. I'd worry about things like getting somewhere on time, finishing tasks, and having too many things to do. I would get easily overwhelmed. I had fears, as well, around being good enough and confident enough and generally a successful person.

HERE ARE SOME THOUGHTS THAT WOULD SPIN IN MY HEAD:

- How will I get everything done?
- Is this really what I want to be doing with my life?
- Am I good enough?
- I should have finished my work.

Later on, I developed a fear of eating things that were not good for me. After making nutritional changes in my life, some confusion arose around what to eat and what not to eat.

I WOULD THINK THINGS LIKE:

- Is this bad for me?
- Am I eating too much?

Now, however, I often watch what I am thinking when I am having a meal or snack and, at times, I catch my head spinning with worried or fearful thoughts.

WHEN I CATCH MYSELF, I RELAX AND CHOOSE TO THINK THOUGHS SUCH AS:

- I am grateful for this meal.
- This tastes really good.

I observe my body to see if I am tense in any areas and consciously relax those muscles.

HERE ARE SOME RECOMMENDED QUESTIONS TO ASK YOURSELF BEFORE OR DURING EATING TO BRING ABOUT AWARENESS:

- Am I really hungry?
- Am I eating out of habit or to satisfy an emotional need?

* What are my thoughts right now?
* Am I feeling at ease?

These are questions to ask pretty regularly to stay in tune with your choices.

Starting now, you can watch what might be patterns of thinking for you around your relationship to food. You may even consider starting a journal to record your answers to these questions, as well as anything else that is troubling you. This might help you in seeing any patterns that you may have. Watch to see what arises. Be your own observer. Observe your thoughts, habits, and feelings around food, and write down what you find.

The most important piece is not to judge yourself for whatever pattern you have developed. The behavior was possibly created because you wanted to find peace. You may have been creating a way to handle what was, and possibly still is, up for you. As an example, food was, to me, a comfort, an emotional ally, when I was feeling emotions I was not equipped to handle. I would look to the food I ate for solace and joy. This pattern of eating for relief was something I did to soothe myself from the pains and challenges I went through. Now, as I watch any of this come up, my "work" is to not judge, but, instead, to love myself.

Whatever it is, watching the behavior is an excellent beginning to the journey of creating a healthy relationship to the wonderful food we ingest.

Be Gentle With Yourself

This journey to health is about exploring and trying new things. Make it fun and easy. There is no need to put pressure on yourself. Being light and easy is an important part of the process. If you come into this with light energy, allowing yourself to do whatever you feel is necessary in each moment without judging or being hard on yourself, you can actually have a good time. For instance, you might be in the process of discovering what foods do not work for you, so you may have stopped eating a bunch of different foods you've been used to eating. As you are going through this process, talk to yourself in a loving, fun way. For instance, if you ate some bread when you were trying not to..."Oh well, no big deal, I'm going to use this as an opportunity to see if there's a reaction."

When I find myself eating something I am not used to or if I am not sure if I will react to a new food, I tell myself positive things and even play with my words. "I am playing with different options seeing what works for me. What a fun process." Or even if I react to something, "Oh well, it's okay. This is temporary."

If you have spent a lifetime pushing, criticizing, and being tough on yourself, this approach may be brand new to you—especially if you catch yourself saying things like, "I can't believe I just ate that. I'm so bad. Why couldn't I have just not eaten that?" and so on. Coming into this with a light energy is one way you can start being gentler with yourself. Also, watch yourself, your thoughts, and your feelings.

Try this: When you notice the thought patterns arising, say to yourself, "Well, there those thoughts are again. How's it going, thoughts?" You don't have to believe them or take them on or you can choose some new ones instead.

HERE ARE SOME EXAMPLES:

- This is a great opportunity to see a pattern I am in.
- This is a great opportunity to try a new food.
- This is a great opportunity to feel ease when I am eating.
- I love myself.
- Everything is going to be okay.

Toss some of these thoughts into your stream of thinking. Just in doing so, you are shifting things. You are recreating your pattern into one based on self-love.

SIMPLIFY FOOD PREPARATION

I love to prepare food, yet I do not like to spend a lot of time doing it. So the main key to my success with food is this: prepare delicious, healthy, simple foods - period. This makes the process of preparing food easy and fun. You can create all kinds of scrumptious meals in only five or ten minutes. This will help you simplify your life.

One way to make preparing food simple is to spend some time in your kitchen cleaning out the refrigerator and cabinets. Look at what you have on the shelves and eliminate foods and condiments that you no longer wish to consume—things like corn syrup, foods that are GMO or not organic, or foods with a lot of refined sugar. This process is transformative, and it is key to making your new lifestyle work for you. For me, I love simplicity and I thrive with easily prepared food.

Now, there are times when a gourmet meal is in order. So I do occasionally invest the time in creating something fantastic and intricate like gluten, dairy, and grain-free pizza, which is one of my favorites. Or I will invite friends over, and each person will take on one piece of the creation.

As I write this book, I am in Mexico. My partner and I did not know what food options we would find here, so we brought with us cacao powder, chia seeds, coconut oil, xylitol, vanilla-flavored stevia, sprouted almond butter, hemp powder, and macadamia nuts. I ate amazing meals today: First, we had a smoothie with spirulina, chlorella, coconut oil, a sweetener, and cacao, with an herbal tea as the base. (I have included a list of superfoods in the section on food lists later in this chapter.) Then, after a workout, we blended some hemp powder, glutamine, vitamin C, and stevia in water for a second smoothie. For lunch, I made seed-based bread, which I ate with almond butter, and was totally satiated. For dinner, I had a simply prepared piece of fish and a salad. These recipes take just a few minutes to make. All you need is the ingredients on hand, a bowl, a pan, some utensils, and a high-quality blender.

If you are used to popping a frozen dinner in the microwave, this may take a little more time to adjust to. But it is worth it! You are worth it!

HEAL THE GUT

There is a strong link between digestive health and psoriasis. Often, healing the gut will help heal the skin. If you are experiencing digestive distress, simple eating is a good choice to make.

SEVERAL THINGS CAN CAUSE DIGESTIVE DISTRESS. SOME ARE:

- Emotional and physical stress
- Leaky gut syndrome (this is when food leaks out of the intestinal wall, causing low absorption of nutrients and increase in absorption of toxins)
- Insufficient good bacteria in the intestines or an imbalance of good and bad bacteria
- Eating foods that you are allergic to or that aggravate your body
- Malnutrition
- An active bacterial, viral, or fungal infection

HERE ARE SOME GOOD EATING GUIDELINES THAT CAN BE HELPFUL IN HEALING THE GUT:

1. Eat easily digested foods. Eat blended smoothies and cooked soups instead of salads for a while. Eventually, salads can be added back in. Raw-food smoothies can be blended in a Vitamix with water or coconut water as a base. You can also blend steamed veggies with water. The recipe for Blended Soup is in the recipe section.
2. Eat veggies lightly steamed or sautéed in coconut oil. This is easy for the body to digest because it is uncomplicated and warm, with only a few ingredients, is soothing, and goes down easily. Coconut oil is anti-microbial and will help if there is any infection active in the body. It's also a medium-chain triglyceride, which is a very easily digested type of fat.
3. Eat excellent-quality food. This means eat non-GMO, organic food as much as you can. The nutrient level of organic food is high, giving lots of good nutrition to our digestive systems. By eating organic food, you are staying away from foods sprayed with pesticides and other chemicals that are harmful to our bodies. Foods that are genetically modified can also be quite harmful to our bodies and have reduced nutrient value.

4. Eat high-quality protein, like wild fish (not farm-raised), 100% grass-fed meat, and wild game if possible. Prepare it simply and make it scrumptious for you. I love to cook my fish in coconut oil with lemon, sea salt and herbs. This is a major staple for me. It provides essential fatty acids and easily digestible protein, keeps my blood sugar balanced, and is also very delicious.

5. Soaked and sprouted nuts and seeds are easy to snack on and to add to meals. I love sprouted almonds with coconut aminos—a coconut-based alternative to soy sauce, dehydrated. You soak most nuts or seeds in water for 4-8 hours and then strain. This begins the sprouting process and makes them much more easily digested. There are enzyme inhibitors on nuts and seeds; soaking them helps to wash these away. You don't want to inhibit the enzymes on the nut or seed, for they are crucial to digesting the food. Some people are sensitive to nuts and seeds and their gut might need more healing before they can digest them. After straining the almonds, add some coconut aminos and dehydrate for a few hours at 105 degrees.

6. Eat foods from the wild, like herbs and flowers. The best place to find such herbs and foods is in the wild, meaning in the woods or in your garden; just be sure they are 100% safe to eat first (not sprayed with pesticides and other herbicides). You can also work with an herbalist or use an herbal guide book to be sure they are safe to ingest. Some farmers' markets and health food stores sell fresh herbs and edible flowers.

7. Drink water with lemon. This stimulates the liver to do a gentle detoxification, is rich in Vitamin C, and has many more benefits.

How you eat is crucial to the healing of your gut, and inevitably also to the healing of psoriasis. Some folks are ultra-sensitive, and eating things that their bodies cannot tolerate wreaks havoc on their systems, causing damage, difficulty assimilating the nutrients that are present, and sometimes also autoimmune conditions.

Digestion is a crucial part of our skin's health. As we take care of our gut, we take care of our whole body, including our skin. Through great self-care around digestion, we begin to see beneficial effects, such as the clearing up of skin problems.

Cleaning Up Your Diet

If you have psoriasis, you may also have a weakened immune system and low energy. Hence, it is very important to eliminate anything that may cause your body extra work or cause it to break down. So, I recommend the elimination diet; basically, you simplify your diet so you're only eating foods that are very easy to digest (see my list below). This is done temporarily to determine which foods help you thrive and which do not. Ideally, this would be done for three months, but I suggest doing it as long as it feels okay for you, and if that is one or two months, that is okay. The elimination diet, means ceasing to eat certain foods that can be inflammatory, then gradually reintroducing them one at a time to see what effect they have.

The food groups to be eliminated are: dairy, gluten, soy, eggs, grains and beans, the nightshades, which include tomatoes, potatoes, and eggplant, and also refined sugars such as brown and white sugar. Beverages include caffeine and alcohol.

After three months of not eating these foods, you may introduce one food back at a time in a small amount—from any of the categories. Consume a small amount at first so that you don't overwhelm your body with something it may reject. It may react more with a larger amount ingested and you might be extra sensitive due to the pure diet you have been on. Then, wait three days to see if there is a reaction. Reactions occur anywhere from right away to three days later, so you need to wait for this long to see what arises.

Look to see if there is any sign of a rash, digestive distress, fogginess or clouded thinking, body pain, headache, sinus problems, or cold symptoms. There could be other symptoms as well.

If there are no symptoms, continue to eat that food, reintroducing it slowly into your diet. Eat it in a small amount and not every day, taking two days off from eating it every week to prevent developing sensitivity to it. I like to take some days off of certain foods that I eat pretty regularly, like coconut oil and chia. I will consciously stop eating them and switch to other oils and proteins like olive oil and wild-caught fish. If you tend to have sensitivities to foods or have allergies, the rotation concept is a good idea. It gives your body a relief from eating the same substance. Play with different recipes and alternate your meals so you are not eating the same foods all the time. When we rotate our foods, we offer our bodies a variety of nutrients.

The process of reintroducing food back into your diet can be done with each food. If there is a reaction, it means it's best not to have that food in your diet and you can eliminate it completely.

So, for example, after you have eliminated all the categories for three months, you may want to start back on dairy. You can try some organic yogurt or raw cheese from a grass-fed animal. Pick one and eat a small amount of it, then notice what happens. Does it give you hives? Digestive distress? Swelling? A tired feeling? You can journal your reactions to keep track of how you feel physically and emotionally for three days after eating the food. If, at the end of a three-day period, you do not notice any negative symptoms, it is likely safe to bring this food back into your diet. Do this by having a small amount of it (in other words, don't eat the entire block of cheese once you decide it's safe for you to eat cheese). If it does give symptoms, then it is likely best to completely eliminate this food from your diet. You can reintroduce it when you feel stronger or healthier, and see how your body reacts then. It is extremely liberating to know if there is something that is wreaking havoc on your body, so you can remove it from your diet.

HERE IS A LIST OF FOODS TO EAT DURING YOUR ELIMINATION TRIAL PERIOD:

* Simple proteins: fish, beef, and wild game. Make sure they are excellent quality. Ideally, the meat should be 100% grass-fed and the fish wild-caught

- All vegetables, including root vegetables such as sweet potato, parsnip and turnip, and squash such as butternut and kabocha
- Berries and fruit, including lemon
- Olive oil or coconut oil. (Be aware that some people can be sensitive to coconut.)
- Soy-free miso
- Seaweed
- Nuts and seeds, including coconut flour, almond flour, and coconut meat
- Xylitol (from the birch tree) or coconut sweetener
- Sea salt

Eat these foods in whatever amounts you like.

I know this way of eating can seem limiting, and that is understandable. But I want you to realize that you can make amazing, delicious dishes from the ingredients that you do well with. I have three days' worth of recipes at the end of my book that I make mostly from the foods on this list, and they are very simple and tasty. Give them a try. Also remember that eliminating foods is temporary. You only need to do this for as long as it takes to discover what foods don't suit you. I think the elimination diet is the best way to find this out, and there are many other books that dive into this more specifically that can guide you. You can also take allergy tests or work with a nutritionist if you would like to go another route to determine which foods to stop eating.

In discovering what foods might not be the best for you, you begin to uncover the foods that help you thrive.

What Works For One Person May Not Work For Another

One piece of the puzzle for finding the foods that work and feel best for you could be found in your blood type. I recommend *Eat Right for Your Blood Type* by Peter J. D'Adamo. For me, realizing that my blood type benefitted from some meat really helped me in healing my body and skin. I was raw and vegan for many years, and when I added wild-caught fish and 100% grass-fed meat into my diet, I began to see improvements in my skin, because, I believe, I am sensitive to grains, which cows are fed if they are not grass-fed. Non-grass-fed cows can also be fed hormones and antibiotics. This fully grass-fed meat feels like healthy medicine for me, offering me crucial nutrients for health and wellness. Eating grass-fed meat, I seem to crave sugar a lot less and feel an evenness and balance within me. I feel more grounded and calm, nourished and fulfilled. Protein provides the body with ample fuel and maintains a healthy blood-sugar level. Sugar is empty calories and does not offer long-term fuel.

I would also like to note that I do not support factory-farmed commercial meat. There are two factors at play here. One is the way the animal is treated. Factory farms often have harsh, awful, very disturbing conditions for animals. I encourage everyone to be aware of this and make his or her decisions accordingly. The second factor is what the animals are fed. They are often fed grains, as mentioned above, at least partially, so if you do not tolerate grains, you may not tolerate eating this meat. Eating meat again was a very difficult decision for me, as I am a huge lover of animals, but I took the advice of some friends and health practitioners and began to eat some fish to start, and meat eventually, in order to consume more protein. I believe that eating some meat helped me nourish myself when a lot of other foods were aggravating my skin. What I like to do before I eat is give thanks to the animal for providing me with food and medicine. Additionally, I do not think it is necessary to eat fish and meat in large amounts.

Ultimately, what I discovered through letting go of different foods in my life is that I thrive when I eat in a balanced way. This means, to me, a variety of foods, eating all of the colors of the rainbow, and some protein, veggies, fruits, nuts, and sweets. I love soups, salads, dips, crackers, seed-based breads, fish, meat, live foods, and cooked foods.

PART 2
NUTRITIONAL GUIDELINES

This section contains some nutritional guidelines to give you a place to begin when choosing what to eat and drink and what to let go of. There are a variety of lists for reference.

I think it is essential to point out that every person is unique and different. You may require something that I didn't suggest for you, and I encourage you to be open to that. These are the foods that helped me in profound ways. This provides a great baseline, and can change your life; however, there may be something you can add or remove that I haven't mentioned.

I list some reference books in the back of my book that guided me into this way of eating. Having tried just about everything in terms of meal plans, I have come to find that the following dietary guidelines have supported me the most thus far. It took many years of experimenting to reach this point.

SUPERFOODS

Superfoods are foods that are jam-packed with vitamins, minerals, and essential nutrients for vibrant living. Including them in your daily life can be extremely helpful to, and can support the creation of, a very healthy environment within and without for a healthy body, mind, and spirit. There are many superfoods to choose from, so it is fun to change them up day to day in your meals and as supplements.

Among the most incredible superfoods are the wild edibles that grow around us. This will vary based on location. They are filled with nutrients that we can only receive from eating wild foods. I feel super-heroine energy when I drink or eat wild edible herbs and flowers. They offer a connection to the wild that we have been removed from in our society that now packages a large proportion of our foods.

I like to add some form of superfood to my meals or snacks. I may add spirulina to a salad dressing or put hemp seeds into a veggie-based noodle dish. You can add edible flowers to just about anything. These are just a few examples of the infinite things you can do to add superfoods to your dishes and drinks.

SOME SUPERFOOD OPTIONS:

- Chia seed
- Hemp seed
- Spirulina
- Chlorella
- Seaweed
- Cacao
- Wild edibles and flowers
- Camu camu
- Lacuma
- Blue-green algae
- Medicinal mushrooms – reishi, cordyceps, chaga
- Coconut
- Goji Berry
- Mulberry
- Bone Broth (Make this only from grass-fed animals. There is a recipe in the book *Practical Paleo*, which I list in the reference section.)

FOODS THAT HEAL:
It is very helpful, though it can take some experimentation, to find the most supportive foods and drinks for you.

HERE IS A LIST OF HEALING FOODS:

Oils: coconut oil, avocado, olive oil

Nuts soaked/sprouted: macadamia nut, almond, hazelnut, pine nut (no need to soak), almond flour (ideally sprouted but okay if not)

Coconut: coconut meat, coconut flour, coconut milk (can be added to soups and smoothies)

Seeds soaked/sprouted: sunflower, chia, pumpkin, hemp (no need to soak), sesame (no need to soak)

Black rice

Miso

Organic starchy root vegetables: sweet potato, squashes, yam, parsnip, turnip, beet

Organic green vegetables: leafy greens galore – there are many options; bok choy, kale, chard, red leaf lettuce, dandelion greens, to name a few – also, broccoli, asparagus, Brussels sprouts, sprouts

Other veggies: cauliflower, cabbage, carrots

Seaweeds: wakame, hijiki, kombu, dulse

Protein: wild meat such as elk and deer, grass-fed meat, wild-caught fish including sardines, pastured chicken and eggs (if you tolerate eggs)

Sweeteners: coconut sugar, stevia (powder or liquid), xylitol (from the birch tree), raw honey (in small amounts)

Organic fruits

Organic, raw, grass-fed dairy: especially butter, can be tolerated by some and may be helpful

Superfoods: such as spirulina, chlorella, blue-green algae

SOME EDIBLE ORAGNIC HERB OPTIONS:

Lambs quarter: lambs quarter is wild spinach, which is high in iron.

Yellow dock: great for healing skin problems.

Wild mint: adds a delicious flavor and can be cooling in the summertime.

Malva: is mucilaginous, which means it has a softening consistency that moistens the mucous membranes. This is great for sinus infections and dry conditions.

Nettles: an anti-histamine that is beneficial for allergies, and high in chlorophyll, so is great for skin and general health.

Lemon balm: has a lemon flavor and is used for calming the nervous system and, as an anti-viral, used for herpes.

Rosemary: can be added to meat and helps with memory.

Basil: a fantastic standard for dips and dressings. It calms the nervous system and is uplifting, easing anxiety

It is important to note that some people may struggle with digesting or tolerating grains, and this is worth experimenting with if you still have stubborn symptoms after eliminating gluten, dairy, sugar, caffeine, alcohol, and eggs. I have noticed that what is called Forbidden Black Rice digests more easily than other grains. It is also very good for your adrenals, along with other black foods such as black beans, black sesame seeds, and some seaweeds. In some cultures it is considered food for royalty.

HERE IS A LIST OF HEALING BEVERAGES:

Water or non-caffeinated tea with fresh lemon added

Fresh water: filtered or spring, such as Mountain Valley Spring Water

Veggie juice: kale, spinach, nettles, cilantro, lemon balm, lemon, etc. you can add some fruit juice if desired: Sometimes citrus can aggravate; in that case, use apple, pear, or other fruit juice.

Coconut water

WHAT TO EAT DURING A BREAKOUT

Any imbalance in your digestive system can aggravate a flare-up on your skin, which is why it's important to eat foods that are easy to digest if you are experiencing an aggravation in the condition of your skin. Our autonomic nervous system has two modes, the parasympathetic and the sympathetic. The sympathetic response occurs when the body is under stress and tells the body that there is imminent harm or fear. The body then shuts down some of its processes, including digestion, so it can handle the stress. So, if you are anxious, you are likely not digesting your food and taking in the nutrients you need for strength and health. If someone has been under stress for a long time, they will have a greater chance of not absorbing or assimilating nutrients from the food they are eating. Stress can create leaky gut and other conditions that could lead to psoriasis. So, the body's digestive system may need repair.

If I am having a flare up—meaning my skin is aggravated—or I am feeling unwell, achy, or disempowered, I use nutrition as a tool for speeding up my healing. What I mean by this is I realize that there is some imbalance in my body, and it is manifesting through my skin or how I feel. Feeling "off" can mean feeling irritable, annoyed, depressed, angry, triggered, sad, insecure, or many other emotions. I use this as an opportunity to play with my daily choices in expediting my healing process from the imbalance. My body is showing me that it is having a tough time, is trying to release something or is under stress. Doing this simple protocol will allow healing to occur and the body to get back on track.

THIS IS WHAT I DO:

1. Eat simply
2. Eat optimum nutrition
3. Choose low sugar and high protein and fats
4. Drink fresh juice
5. Eat blended meals, smoothies, or veggie broth
6. Meditate
7. Eat wild fish and greens once per day
8. Eat light meals
9. Do a short fast, for less than 24 hours
10. Eat only when I'm feeling good

HERE ARE THE STEPS FOR A SHORT FAST:

1. Eat an early dinner at 5 pm and stop eating after that. Drink tea, broth, juice, and lemon in water from 5 pm on but do not consume solid food.
2. The following morning, drink any of the liquids listed above, in the List of Healing Beverages.
3. Then, around 1 pm, eat one of the following: a smoothie with fruit and leafy greens, (for instance: one banana, one apple, filtered water, and a handful of leafy greens), blended soup from my recipe section, or a piece of fruit.
4. Eat dinner at 5 or 6 pm using any recipe in my recipe section, such as "Delish Fish" or "Veggies and Protein for Clear Skin". You can skip step 3 if desired.

I create delicious meals and make sure that my taste buds are singing and happy. Find the meals that really satisfy you *and* are uncomplicated during a flare-up. It is very important to eat food that is as easy as possible to digest if you are going through aggravation of any sort.

HERE ARE SOME EXAMPLES OF EASY-TO-DIGEST FOODS:

1. Fish works well, especially a light white fish like turbot or cod that is wild-caught. I know it works for me because, after I eat it, I feel balanced and nourished.
2. Simple smoothies with banana and greens, veggies with coconut or olive oil, a piece of fruit, mashed avocado with banana, or a cup of herbal tea.
3. From my recipe section at the end of the book, try "Blended Soup for Clear Skin", "Chia Cereal", "Super Sauté", "Vibrant Skin Salad", or "Butternut Cream".

Even when you're not having a flare-up, it is always best to eat while feeling good, aligned, and at peace. This means, no matter what you're eating, stay calm and at ease, not agitated or distressed, during the meal. This will shift the nervous system into parasympathetic mode, which makes it easy for your body to digest and absorb its food.

One way to do this is by asking yourself how you feel about eating a particular food or meal. If you feel at ease and good about it, eat on. If you are feeling off, frustrated, angry, or stressed, then I would suggest waiting until you find your center to have a meal. If you are feeling off, then this is a great chance to find your way back to peace. You can practice getting aligned, which we will address more in Chapter Seven. If you are hungry or need the food for strength and/or nourishment, I would suggest eating something simple such as a smoothie or a piece of fruit.

FOODS AND DRINKS THAT MAY BE AGGRAVATING:

After following the elimination diet for a period of time, refer to these lists. There is a lot of overlap between the first two lists and the elimination diet. The list of foods and drinks not to ingest can seem overwhelming at first, I know, but I can tell you that eliminating these foods from my diet has helped me clear my skin, lift my spirits, heal many diseases, and be calmer and happier. If you are eating foods that are hard for your body to process or that you are simply allergic to, it can create disease in your body. This is just a guide to begin with and it may not be your nutritional solution. It's all about perspective. If you think the thought, *It is difficult to let go of gluten,* then it may be difficult. If you think the thought, *It will be smooth and easy and exciting to let go of gluten,* then it can be just that. Glutinous foods can cause some people a variety of health challenges including skin problems, body aches and pains, digestive distress, foggy thinking, depression, and more. After eliminating gluten and some other foods you may begin to notice better, clearer, more radiant skin. Among other positive effects you might notice are better energy, better digestion, feeling more peace, and fewer headaches, colds and flus.

In general, there are certain foods that may be aggravators for you. The list below provides guidelines to experiment with and find out what foods you can tolerate. I stay away from all of these because I have found that they may aggravate my skin and me. I am totally content and at peace with this choice. Again, what does and does not work for you may be totally different. This is only a base guide, to be used as a gauge going forward. What I have come to understand through this process is that it may not be only what I eat that is aggravating me; it may also be how I feel about what I eat. It's only after twenty years of working on altering my daily intake of food that I realized this. I continue to eat from the "Foods that Heal" list that appears earlier in this chapter most of the time because I have grown accustomed to it, and I am at ease with this choice; I also know that this ease assists with the food's nutritional assimilation and value in my body.

FOODS THAT MAY AGGRAVATE:

- Hydrogenated and vegetable oils such as soy and margarine
- Common allergens such as eggs, dairy, gluten, corn, soy
- Refined sugar and high glycemic sugars e.g., high fructose corn syrup, or white sugar
- Iodized salt
- Heated chocolate e.g., chocolate bars and hot chocolate that are not raw (heating chocolate increases caffeine content and destroys some nutrients)
- Citrus
- Tomatoes
- Nightshades including white potatoes, tomatoes, peppers and eggplant
- White rice
- Grains

DRINKS THAT MAY AGGRAVATE:

- Coffee
- Alcohol
- Sugary fruit juice
- Soda
- Anything with food colorings or synthetic preservatives

SUBSTITUTES FOR FOODS THAT MAY AGGRAVATE

One of my most amazing tips, that I am excited to share, is that there is always a healthy, wonderful food that you can substitute for something that is not working for you. Giving foods and lifestyle habits up can actually be easier than you think. What I suggest is that you find substitutes and adjust your choices to make them work for you. This can help you in shifting your ways of eating.

For instance, if you are giving up refined sugar, you can add in substitutes such as xylitol or fresh fruit more often; adjust your lifestyle by eating more protein, which helps with cravings by fulfilling your body's need for nourishment and stabilizes blood sugar, or consider using supplements that can help cut down on cravings for refined sugar, such as hemp protein, cinnamon, and chromium.

FOOD SUBSTITUTE LIST:

Eggs: Chia seed, soaked, is a great egg substitute to use in making breads and cookies; Irish moss (a seaweed), when it is soaked for at least six hours, strained and blended with water, can act like an egg in a recipe. It can fluff up breads, cookies, and many other meal options.

Wheat and grain breads: Coconut flour or almond flour breads; lettuce, cabbage, or nori as a wrap

Pasta: Kelp noodles; spiral noodles you can make yourself from squash, zucchini, or other veggies

Sugar: Xylitol; coconut sugar, stevia (powder or liquid), raw honey (in small amounts)

Canola, soy, and other veggie oils: Coconut; olive, raw butter (from grass-fed animals), hemp oil

Cheese: Nut or seed cheese, such as macadamia nut or sunflower seed cheese, nutritional yeast with olive oil and sea salt

Cookies or cake: Desserts from coconut flour or almond flour with xylitol (100% birch) or coconut sugar

Desserts: "Banana Pudding" or "Chocolate Cookie Dough for Clear Skin" (in the recipe section in the back of this book)

Soda and drinks with aspartame or corn syrup: Fresh veggie juice with lots of lemon; lemon water, herbal water

Cooked or heated chocolate: Raw chocolate. (My favorite brand is Lulu's)

Salad dressing: Olive oil, lemon, and sea salt. Blend in avocado, nuts or seeds, or zucchini to make it creamy

Chips: Jilz Crackers are like chips and are delicious and great for food sensitive people; pea chips; cucumbers; sliced veggies with coconut oil and sea salt, dehydrated for a few hours, Jackson's Honest Sweet Potato Chips

Ice cream: Coconut milk ice cream

Mayonnaise: Avocado

The list of foods you can eat is long, and you will be amazed at the incredible options you have within this list to create some delicious meals. Try just one of these options or many. Some people may need to alter this a bit if they are sensitive to nuts and/or seeds.

There are endless options for replacing the foods that you are eliminating. Remembering this is key in helping you successfully navigate this stage of elimination and integrate new foods into your life. Ideally, you will eventually fall in love with what you eat, as you develop a taste for these different foods—especially because of how eating this way can make you feel.

PART 3
USING SUPPLEMENTS AND HERBS FOR HEALING

THE NEXT APPROACH TO HEALING THAT WE'LL LOOK AT IN THE PHYSICAL REALM IS USING SUPPLEMENTS AND HERBS.

SOME THINGS YOU CAN DO WITH YOUR IMMUNE SYSTEM AND INFLAMMATION INCLUDE:

1. Take medicinal mushrooms daily to modulate the immune system.
2. Exercise for short periods of time instead of long. Long workouts can be a stressor for certain people. Short workouts give your body ample recovery time.
3. Take turmeric capsules. Turmeric is anti-inflammatory and rich in antioxidants.
4. Eat plenty of leafy greens. They are high in chlorophyll and minerals, such as calcium and magnesium, iron, vitamin C, beta-carotene, and protein, with all essential amino acids. Chlorophyll oxygenates the cells, strengthens the immune system, lowers the effects of pollution, lowers inflammation, and helps with psoriasis, eczema, and acne.
5. Take vitamins D3. It is an immune modulator and sometimes those with autoimmune conditions can be deficient in this important vitamin.
6. Take probiotics. Healthy bacteria balance the bacteria in the gut, and help create a strong immune system.
7. Take Chinese Mountain Ant. It is one of the highest sources of zinc, which is classically known to help with acne and the skin. This is great for psoriasis because it helps fortify a weak immune system and modifies an overactive system.
8. Drink a veggie juice regularly. This is deeply hydrating on a cellular level and offers nourishment and balance to the body.

9. Consume coconut oil. Coconut oil is great for psoriasis because it addresses the immune system as it has anti-microbial, anti-fungal, anti-viral, and anti-bacterial, qualities; it also contains medium-chain fatty acids, so it is effective against colds, flu, and candida. It is high in caprylic acid, so it is an effective anti-fungal, and it increases the white blood cell count.

As I mentioned earlier, often those with psoriasis have digestive systems that need healing and getting on a regimen that includes certain supplements such as probiotics, digestive enzymes, and glutamine is helpful.

HERE ARE SOME SUPPLEMENTS THAT CAN ASSIST THE DIGESTIVE SYSTEM:

1. Since people with psoriasis often have hidden (or sometimes obvious) food allergies or sensitivities, take a digestive enzyme on an empty stomach first thing in the morning. This helps eat up many of the floating allergens or unneeded food particles in the system. Digestive enzymes work as an anti-inflammatory when taken on an empty stomach as well. Also, take an enzyme with each meal to help digest your food.
2. Take a probiotic. Make sure it is great quality. I suggest some brands in the reference section at the end of the book. You want your probiotics to have at least 10 billion cells. I take one with 25 billion cells. I also check that they are gluten and dairy free, and that any additives are minimal, for instance containing only the vegetable capsule, not extra unnecessary ingredients like citric acid or magnesium stearate. I have grown to trust certain brands as actually containing what they say they do in their product, and know them to be trustworthy companies of high integrity and intention. Probiotics are crucial for the immune system since immune system health begins in the digestive system when you have enough probiotic cells in proportion to harmful bacteria.

3. Take glutamine. Some people cannot tolerate this, so start with a small amount and see how you feel. If you cannot tolerate glutamine, you may have some diarrhea. It has been said that if you are sensitive to MSG, you may have a sensitivity or allergic reaction to glutamine. I personally have not experienced this and have had excellent results. Glutamine repairs the intestinal wall. There will possibly be damage, literally holes in the intestines that need repair. Glutamine fills in these holes, lining the intestines. It can also be very soothing and relieving when you are feeling any pain or soreness in the tummy. Repair of the intestines is an important piece to healing the gut.

4. Chia seeds offer a great quality essential fatty acid and good fiber. Also considered a superfood, chia seed is great for helping the bowels stay regular. It can even work for some people after one usage to give them a well-formed bowel movement. It is an alternative to conventional cereals and puddings, offering a mucilaginous consistency when sprouted in water.

5. Often with skin diseases, there can be a lot of candida present. Candida occurs naturally in the body. An overgrowth occurs in some folks for multiple reasons and it causes a condition known as candidiasis. Then there can be some symptoms such as skin problems and much more. Anti-fungal herbs such as Pau d'arco and Oregon grape root can be helpful, as well as an anti-candida diet. The diet suggests low sugar and high-quality protein and veggies as the basis.

6. Colostrum, an immune-enhancing supplement, is a key component to breast milk, and is something you can purchase at a health-food store (it is usually sourced from cows and does not contain breast milk). Some people who were not breastfed could have psoriasis or other conditions from not being fed the immune- and digestion-building nutrients in breast milk. Just by increasing some nourishing foods and superfoods, you will receive many of the nutrients you may be lacking.

7. High-quality oils, such as coconut oil, fermented cod liver oil, good quality fish oil, krill oil, grass-fed butter (if you can tolerate dairy), cacao butter, olive oil, and hemp oil work to keep inflammation down. They give the body the essential fats needed to protect the nervous system and feed the skin. For skin, especially, evening primrose oil –an essential fatty acid source rich in GLA (gamma-linoleic-acid) – encourages health. I have seen excellent results with eczema with this oil.

8. Stress is a big component of psoriasis, so it's essential to focus on that. Supplements for stress relief for psoriasis may include B vitamins and herbs such as motherwort, oatstraw, and tulsi. Rescue Remedy, a flower essence from the company Bach, is one remedy specifically formulated for stress, trauma, and anxiety. Rescue Remedy contains five individual flower essences mixed together. Bach Flower Essences are the ones you will find in most health food stores, such as Whole Foods, though there are other good brands, such as FES. Flower essences are extractions of flowers that help on the emotional plane and give effective assistance when working in areas where someone may feel stuck and frustrated. Bach has many other individual essences as well. They work very specifically with emotions such as despair, jealousy, or anger. Elm is for overwhelm, Larch for confidence, and White Chestnut for calming a worried mind, for example. They help with specific patterns and tendencies like fear of public speaking or inability to make decisions. Reishi is a medicinal mushroom that can be extremely calming to our spirit. L-theanine is an amino acid that is taken for mental clarity and staying calm and centered.

9. It is very helpful to begin a practice of keeping your body moving, doing healthy exercise of some sort. This helps if you are undergoing stress by processing your tension and letting it move through you. Exercise often gets you in touch with your body so that you begin paying more attention to your breathing. It also provides your body with a healthy flow of oxygen and blood.

Exercise helps release healthy hormones, such as endorphins, in your body, which help you to feel good. Sweating is also helpful because it releases toxins. I encourage finding something that you love doing that moves your body and adding it into your daily or weekly schedule. Perhaps it's taking a walk for ten minutes, or you may choose dancing, hiking, Qigong, yoga, biking, swimming, or going to the gym.

10. Nascent iodine has helped keep my skin clear. It is a type of iodine that is found in liquid form and is very easily absorbed in the body. It is considered a more safe and useful source of iodine than potassium iodine. It supports the thyroid and helps with nutrient absorption and detoxification. I have noticed that my skin will clear during a breakout more quickly when I add this type of iodine into my regimen.

11. Sunlight can be very helpful for psoriasis in small doses, as it stimulates vitamin-D production in the body, and those with psoriasis may be low in this vitamin. Vitamin D can be taken internally as well.

12. Essential Oils – Smelling calming essential oils, like lavender and orange, is a wonderful way to uplift the spirit and feel good in your body.

13. Some medical options include non-steroidal anti-inflammatory drugs, corticosteroids, and antidepressants. I prefer the holistic route to healing as much as possible and encourage others to do the same. But there are times when these medications can be helpful and supportive, and even necessary.

Remember, in supplements, it is important to have as few extra ingredients, such as fillers and additives, as possible. The helpfulness of herbs and supplements is always specific to the individual and the causes of their psoriasis. It is important to customize herbs, flower essences, and supplements for your particular needs. You can work on this with your practitioner; if you do not have one, maybe it is time to find one. My favorite way to find a practitioner is by word of mouth, through a friend or someone who has had experience working with a particular person. You can also do some online searching or check with local holistic schools or health-food stores for suggestions.

It is helpful to find someone who works with nutrition, herbs, allergy testing, and other modalities such as acupuncture if those are things you would like to explore. Look for a practitioner with multiple skills; you may discover that it is helpful to have a couple of practitioners to work with.

I am available for personalized consultations, which can be scheduled at my website, skinsoulutions.com.

TOPICAL OPTIONS FOR HEALING SKIN

Topical options include capsaicin, aloe, coconut oil, and shea butter. Derma E has a product called Psorzema that can offer excellent relief for itchy skin and can help remove dry flakiness. Sunlight, as mentioned above, can be helpful and has been shown to help clear psoriasis.

Herbal Tea Poultice

I like to make a strong batch of healing herbal tea to put on my skin. You do this by letting the tea steep overnight, or for at least eight hours. Then strain. Then, using a soft cloth saturated with the tea, lay it on your skin where the psoriasis is present.

My favorite teas to use are burdock root and Oregon grape root. Boil the tea briefly and then let it simmer for at least 20 minutes, to get the essential constituents out of the herbs. Make sure the tea has cooled down before applying topically. You can get these herbs in bulk at a health-food store, online, or you may have an herbal apothecary close to you. I mention some options in my reference section.

Simple Water Therapy

Another very helpful tool is water therapy. End your shower with about ten seconds of very cold water, or you can alternate hot and cold throughout the shower. This is very stimulating for the nervous system. Circulation of the blood increases when the skin is exposed to very cold water, and the body's immune defenses are aroused and stimulated to protect the body from harm and disease.

Soap-Free

It could help to stop using soap on psoriasis as it can irritate the psoriasis. You could use just water, or a gentle scrub made from salt or sugar, essential oils, and oils like jojoba or olive oil. You can purchase one or make your own. Salt can also be aggravating and too aggressive, yet may work for some if used with a gentle scrubbing action.

Medical Treatments

Common topical medical treatments include topical steroids or coal tar. There is also a vitamin D analog cream called calcipotreine, which is another useful treatment. Sterol anti-inflammatories are injected directly onto the plaques to help them to subside. The cortisone creams that you can get at a pharmacy can be helpful for very itchy situations that need relief. They can help prevent scratching, which often exacerbates the situation.

HERBAL SUPPORT

Since many of you may not be familiar with herbs, I will talk now about some herbs that can help from multiple perspectives, including stress and liver support. This will give you some options to help you determine how best to approach your issues.

HERBS FOR THE NERVOUS SYSTEM

The nervous system is aggravated by stress and anxiety. Stress impacts the body for different people in different ways. Stress will likely be reflected on the skin of people who tend to have psoriasis or other skin issues.

Herbs that are good for the nervous system include oatstraw, passionflower, and motherwort. Below, I have described each one and some of its properties.

Oatstraw

The Latin name for oatstraw is *Avena sativa*. Avena means "nourishing" in Latin. The stem is a mood elevator, a nervine, a nervous-system tonic, a nutritive, a rejuvenative, and a restorative herb. It treats anxiety, depression, emotional distress, nervousness, nervous breakdown, post-traumatic stress disorder, and much more. Topically, as a poultice, it relieves itching related to eczema or psoriasis. It is very high in minerals and vitamins, so it is extremely nutritious and supportive of a taxed system that needs some nourishment.

Passionflower

The Latin name for passionflower is *Passiflora incarnate*. It is effective for emotional stress and to help relax an over-thinking mind that is spinning with thoughts. It relaxes the nerves and calms the spirit, heart, liver, and central nervous system. It induces rest and helps aid in sleep for those that are under stress. The tea is also helpful for anger, depression, irritability, restlessness, hysteria, and worry. But use this herb in moderation, as large doses may cause vomiting and nausea.

Motherwort

The Latin name for motherwort is *Leonurus cardiaca*. Motherwort calms anxiety and stress that may contribute to heart problems. It also helps with nervous exhaustion, insomnia, panic attacks, heartbreak, hot flashes, depression (including postpartum and bipolar), hysteria, melancholy, insomnia, restlessness, shingles, heart palpitations, pre-menstrual syndrome, skin hypersensitivity, herpes, and much more. Taking motherwort is like getting a hug from your mother. It can uplift mothers and help those who are overly nurturing and motherly to let go. It is important to avoid it in cases of excessive menstrual bleeding. Also avoid during pregnancy.

HERBS FOR SKIN AND LIVER

There is a direct correlation between the ability of the liver to process toxins and hormones, and the health of the skin. Here are some great herbs for the skin and liver that can be taken as a tea, tincture, or capsule: milk thistle, dandelion (leaf and root), burdock root, Oregon grape root, and red clover.

Milk Thistle

The Latin name for milk thistle is *Sylybum marianum*. Milk thistle seed helps protect the liver, prevent toxins from entering the interior of liver cells, and detox the liver. Milk thistle improves the liver's function and helps promote the growth of healthy liver cells. It treats bile-duct inflammation, hepatitis, and depression. Milk Thistle is a common herb used to help those with psoriasis because of its ability to reduce inflammation, slow down excessive cell growth, aid in detoxification, and support the liver's function.

Dandelion

The Latin name for dandelion is *Taraxacum officinale.* Dandelion is a blood purifier, assisting in filtering and straining wastes from the blood. The root improves the metabolism of fat, helping in some cases of psoriasis, where the person has a hard time with digesting and processing fats. The root is high in calcium, iron, zinc, choline, pectin, and much more. It can help heal psoriasis as well as eczema, depression, and candida. The leaf is high in B1, B2, folic acid, calcium, and phosphorus. The leaf as a food and the root tea have a very highly bitter flavor, and adding this bitter element into the diet can aid in digestion, helping to increase the secretion of digestive juices. In Ayurvedic medicine, the bitter flavor is known to break up congestion in the liver and relieve itchy skin conditions. Dandelion helps release stored emotions of anger and fear.

Burdock

The Latin name for burdock root is *Arctium lappa*. It helps detoxify the body of wastes through the liver, kidneys, lymph system, large intestines, lungs, and skin. It is anti-inflammatory and anti-fungal. It is a treatment for psoriasis, eczema, and acne. The root is rich in calcium, iron, vitamin C, and zinc. The seed is high in essential fatty acids. You can make a tea of the root or leaf and add other herbs such as dandelion root and Oregon grape root for a great blend for the skin. Take burdock root internally as well as topically. If using it externally, let it cool, make a compress, and put it on the psoriasis for relief and healing. You can also add the tea to your bathtub. I love adding burdock root to my soups.

Oregon Grape Root

The Latin name for Oregon grape root is *Mahonia aquifolium*. Topically, it can help slow the excessive production of skin cells that occurs with psoriasis. Oregon grape has a constituent called berberine that helps fight bacterial and fungal infections. It also treats acne, eczema, staph, and herpes. Use it internally and externally. The flower essence could help someone with psoriasis, because it is used to treat self-criticism and helps you to love and accept yourself. Avoid in pregnancy, hyperthyroid conditions, and in cases of excessive gas.

Red Clover

The Latin name for red clover is *Trifolium pretense*. Red clover is a blood cleanser that targets the skin. It helps in detoxification, and is deeply nutritive. It contains protein, calcium, B vitamins, selenium, copper, iron, and chromium. It is also a lymphatic mover. It helps many conditions including psoriasis, acne and eczema. Use it topically or internally for psoriasis. It could be very helpful for those with psoriasis as a flower essence because it brings calm in the face of fear. Do not use during pregnancy.

There are always possibilities for allergic reactions to herbs. Please take this into consideration when using any of these herbs and consult a doctor and/or practitioner before use. There are contraindications in certain circumstances, so look into this before beginning any herbal regimen.

Now that we have covered the physical aspect of healing your skin, we will begin discussing the emotional component.

CHAPTER 5
Emotional Healing

∗ ∗ ∗

CLEARING PSORIASIS IS AS MUCH an outside job as it is an inside one. By focusing on the physical realm—our nutrition and lifestyle—we may see some healing of our psoriasis. But to really go all the way with our healing, we must look within. Now it is time to take a deeper look at our emotional lives and see ways we may be able to heal. In this chapter, we will look at the patterns and behaviors we live by. There, we may discover the obstacles keeping us from moving forward in life.

There are four fundamentals to the emotional component which will help encourage the healing of your skin.

THESE FUNDAMENTALS INCLUDE:

1. Developing a genuine, deep love for yourself.
2. Allowing yourself to fully feel your feelings.
3. Taking responsibility for your own feelings.
4. Realizing that your feelings help to manifest your reality.

It is truly an art, healing your body.

1. DEVELOP A GENUINE, DEEP LOVE FOR YOURSELF

Then, you can take this a step further and love yourself in the face of the pain that arises for you. There is no better person in the world to love deeply than yourself.

"Neurons that fire together wire together. You can rewire your brain for higher consciousness by focusing on love."

—Deepak Chopra

Loving oneself is a journey, especially if you have spent most of your life being hard on yourself, critical, or beating yourself up. Know that just acknowledging that you have not loved yourself is a gigantic step. Now, this may not even be an issue for some folks. You may already love yourself as you are, but doing these steps is a good practice regardless.

There are four steps I have taken to love myself. These steps have worked for me, and I offer them to you, as they may give you some help in your process.

Step One: Acknowledge the part of yourself that has been hard on you for so long. In just bringing awareness and light to that harsh or critical part of yourself, you offer yourself the chance to be non-judgmental and kind and grant yourself love in the process.

Step Two: Spend some time acknowledging where you learned this way of being. There may have been many factors contributing to a lack of self-appreciation.

- It may have been all that you witnessed growing up.
- Maybe you were in a very competitive situation at school or at home.
- You may have grown up not eating nourishing food that met your desires and needs.
- You may have judged yourself.
- You may have been judged.
- You may have not been supported in loving and appreciating yourself.
- You may have been subjected to a lot of television or other media that encourages comparison with others and teaches us that we are not enough as we are.

Step Three: Be softer with yourself. Once you can see where this pattern of not loving yourself developed, you can bring in a loving, soft energy to this area of your life. Make a choice to learn to love yourself as you are right now. Affirm it by writing it down and stating it out loud. "I love myself as I am." Continue to watch the self-deprecating thoughts that arise—and just allow them. Even though that may sound counter-intuitive, allowing them will give them room to come up and go out, rather than fighting them and giving them more power, or suppressing them. The more you watch the thoughts, feelings, and actions that arise out of not loving yourself, the closer you are to truly loving yourself. Then, from this place of allowing, start to introduce thoughts that feel good.

SOME EXAMPLES OF SELF-LOVING THOUGHTS ARE AS FOLLOWS:

* I love myself.
* I am great just as I am.
* I love how kind, fun, loving, sincere, big-hearted, conscientious I am.
* I am enjoying myself.

It may be that another phrase offers you the same peace. This process instantly offers relief and peace in the face of challenging situations. This is true self-care.

HERE ARE A COUPLE OF QUESTIONS TO ASK YOURSELF:

* Can I love myself even when I am afraid, even when circumstances are happening that I cannot control and a lot of emotions come up for me, such as fear, anger, frustration, and being overwhelmed?
* Can I offer myself compassion, empathy, and deep appreciation, as I am, right now?
* One gift of having skin challenges is that it gives you the opportunity to see where you need to find love and appreciation of who you are. It asks you to fine-tune your life in many ways.

Step Four: Discover your own worth.

"If you realized how beautiful you are,
you would fall at your own feet."

—Byron Katie

You are worthy just as you are now. Your mind may try to fight this with criticism, or try to motivate you to improve in some way by nitpicking or putting you down. But if you can sit with this and start to see the truth in it, this will go a long way toward helping you love yourself. Once you find your value and worthiness then you have found self-love.

If coming to the truth of your own worthiness is not something you're ready for, here are small steps you can take to get there:

At the end of each day, sit down and reflect on the wonderful things you did and felt in that day, seeing all that you do as having value. This can include making a good meal, spending time with your kids, your pet or your family, or doing whatever work you do. Find the value in it, with or without other people expressing their appreciation. Write down how you value yourself or go over a list in the morning in bed or right before your sleep. It has value even if it is seemingly a small act, like offering a smile to someone, seeing yourself choose something that is good for you, or watching yourself do something different in a tough situation.

HERE ARE SOME EXAMPLES OF WHAT YOU CAN SAY TO YOURSELF:

- I value the time I spent helping others today.
- I appreciate myself for putting so much great energy into my work today.
- I love that I ate intuitively at lunch.
- I really see how I relaxed the muscles in my jaw instead of clenching them when I was upset. This helped me ease my stressful feelings.

* I watched my thoughts when I was in line at the grocery store. I just noticed how frustrated I was and didn't focus on it.
* I see how I focused on the good in my friend.
* I love how I felt in the clothes I chose to wear today. I looked good too.

Be the observer of your mind trying to criticize, and just witness it, without judgment. Upon observing this, send yourself some love. When you catch yourself in this self-criticism, you may notice a feeling in your body that is heavy, or your muscles may be tight. Just notice this and send it love and see if the sensations soften. You will begin to see that you are worthy of great love; you loving you, no matter what.

Use an affirmation regularly. One of my favorite affirmations is: I am worthy. I love sitting with the word itself, worth, and letting it seep into my consciousness and my cells. I feel such a profound sense of peace and calmness when I feel what worthiness feels like in the body. It is helpful to tap into the feeling that goes along with each affirmation. Really feel that you are worthy, kind, conscientious, thoughtful, loving. The feeling is what creates more of the same.

I spent the majority of my life with low self-esteem, not realizing the immense value I had to contribute and offer to this world. I remember growing up feeling confused and uncertain about everything that was happening in my life. As I mentioned earlier, I could not figure out how to handle all of the emotions that arose within me, and I felt that I did not fit in.

I spent ages fifteen through thirty-eight being "boy crazy." I defined my value by their appreciation and love for me. After a very dramatic, intense relationship ended, I decided it was time to focus on myself, and I began to look within for appreciation, value, and love. After years of cultivating this love within myself, I started seeing a man who has grown to become an incredible reflection and teacher. Being with him, I have grown by leaps and bounds. He has supported me in my power, so I have found myself comfortable with being powerful. He has inspired me to take responsibility for my choices and life. He has helped me to accept more than react, to trust and appreciate more instead of be jealous, and to see myself instead of wait for another to see me. I moved from relying on others for empowerment to finding it within. Once I realized how much I have to offer and teach, I then began to find my self-worth.

You may, like me, have spent your life not knowing what loving yourself really means. We aren't given much guidance in school on this topic. And there may have been circumstances, or even your skin condition, that blocked you from seeing yourself as the fabulous person that you are.

EXERCISES FOR LOVING YOURSELF:
Here are some simple exercises for growing in love with you. I suggest picking one exercise at a time. You could chose a different one each day or each week and just play with it.

1. To start, find the places you feel imperfect, less than you would like to be, and just be aware of them. For instance, where in your life do you feel like you have negative thoughts and energy? Notice where in your life you are judging yourself or talking to yourself in a way that is harsh or hateful. All you need to do is see this when it arises. Then, do nothing. Do not judge the judgment. Just see that this is something you are doing and, possibly, have done for a very long time. It may be habitual at this point.
2. Meditate on loving mantras and words, for example:
   * I am worthy.
   * I am at peace.
   * I feel joy.
3. Do what you love. What do you love? Sometimes the best way to figure out what you love is by knowing what you do not love. Write a list of what you do not love and then write a list of what you do love. What you do not love can include anything. It can be an emotion, a circumstance, a condition--basically whatever does not feel good. Then, do what you love as much as you can.
4. Look at the psoriasis on your body with loving energy instead of anger. This may be challenging when you are so pissed off that

you have this disease on your body. Maybe just start off by imagining that you are sending it loving energy. Then, touch it with your eyes closed and say to yourself, "I see you and love you" or "I'm here. Everything is going to be okay." Then, try this with your eyes open.

5. Notice whatever emotions you may be experiencing right now. Allow what comes up to be, no matter what. Just let it be.

6. Similar to the list above of the ways you value what you did in the day, write a list of all the qualities you love about yourself. It could be as simple as "I love my hair" or "I feel good when I take a bath".

MAKE A LIST AND HAVE FUN WITH IT:

* I love my feet.
* I love how kind I am to animals.
* I love how generous I am.

Just sit and write down all the things you can think of. It may be just one thing that you loved about yourself that day. That is fine.

With these tools as go-tos, you can now begin practicing some new practices to love yourself.

> *"Love is a state of Being. Your love is not outside; it is deep within you. You can never lose it, and it cannot leave you. It is not dependent on some other body, some external form."*

> —ECKHART TOLLE

2. ALLOW YOURSELF TO FULLY FEEL YOUR EMOTIONS

When I was young, I struggled with my emotions. Now, however, I find myself embracing life's challenges, allowing its difficulties, and seeing deep emotions that arise as an opportunity to fully feel the experience of life. Life is magnificent, and feeling the different emotions in your body and being present with them is a wonderful skill to develop. I find the swell of tears to be a huge release and almost pleasurable. But all these skills that I have developed took time and practice. I used to ignore and suppress a lot of emotions, afraid of their potency. Allowing emotions is about not resisting what arises, and even embracing them. I had a pattern for years of deadening my emotions, avoiding them, ignoring them, and repressing them for fear of feeling pain and discomfort. I just did not have the capacity to handle the intense emotions.

I encourage those with psoriasis to see if there is a support group in their area or start one. It may be very helpful and supportive to have people you can share with and also listen to. You can gain much insight and relief when you are honest about your pain and hear about the pain of others.

When I went back to Pittsburgh, right around when my psoriasis healed, to help my family move out of the house we grew up in, I knew this would be big for me emotionally, and I was absolutely right; it was. I worked very hard moving and helping my family. Well, a great deal happened on that trip that, earlier in my life, would have put me into bed, literally sick or with a major skin breakout. This is a recurring pattern I have had since a kid; that I could not handle everything around me. I was sick a lot and had skin issues, and I see now that I was overwhelmed with all the emotional suppression that had become a habit for me. When I went home this time, I recognized that uncomfortable feelings were alive for me. (I use the word "alive" throughout this book in a way suggested by Marshall Rosenberg in his book *Nonviolent Communication: A Language of Life* to mean what is at the forefront of the mind, or is the most predominant emotion in the moment.) A lot of it stemmed from handling the emotions around moving out of the house I grew up in and seeing that this would be a new phase of life. There were also some challenging family dynamics, because everyone was under stress, which was hard to handle emotionally. My muscles were constricted a lot due to this. I was tense, and my body was in fight or flight mode much of the time.

During the move, I took breaks and spent time practicing, very intentionally, being with the emotions. I did so, and I realized that it was a lot for me to deal with, and I ended up really processing it on my way back to Colorado. Swells of emotions began to arise when I was on the plane. I just allowed them and wept, and they passed with sweet release.

I feel relief and sometimes even joy when I allow my emotions to be and come up and out. It feels wonderful not to resist what comes up; to witness myself in my depth of feeling.

So, as I was crying on the plane, I consciously realized that I cannot control what anybody chooses. I can most definitely be connected within myself continually and control what I choose. I cannot change my family or any person, yet I can change my energy and what I choose to do with it. This was revolutionary for me. I am my own person and have my own journey through life. I see this as a chance, an opportunity, to grow and become more adept at staying centered during challenge and hardship. If I can also love and accept others and feel my emotions, then I am successful in many ways. I am successful at focusing on my energy field and not theirs. I am successful at allowing them to be and accepting them fully as they are. I am successful in allowing deep emotions to arise and be with—not resist—those emotions. This creates a perfect foundation for growth and transformation, as well as peace amid chaos.

Emotions are magnetic, charged with a feeling that lights up something within you. Each one carries a resonance of its own. Some are harder to feel than others. They may actually feel painful or heavy in the body, in the tissues, yet once allowed, you may notice that the pain subsides and disappears, and a light feeling in your body ensues. Other emotions feel so juicy and brightening, they ignite your senses and open your heart.

As I mentioned early in the book, just a short while before I developed psoriasis, I was bulimic. I was bulimic for part of high school and the first year of college. One day, I woke up and saw that I was really harming myself, and I knew I had to stop this pattern of binging and purging. So I stopped. Not everyone can just stop bulimia cold turkey like that. Again, it is very helpful to find support and guidance during the process. I had become bulimic in an attempt to gain some control in a world where so much was happening that was out of my control. I knew I was beautiful, but I believed I had to maintain that in order to survive and be seen in the world. My physical appearance was all I thought I had to offer. Also, as I mentioned earlier, I ate emotionally, meaning when I felt an emotion I could not handle, I chose to eat instead because it seemed to temporarily take away my pain. (I did that with alcohol as well.) So, if a difficult emotion, like fear, anger, or sadness, arose for me, I often looked to binging to find pleasure and move away from the perceived pain and fear of my emotions, and then would purge to maintain control. At that time, I was really suffering and wanted to find some security.

Learning to handle and fully allow emotions is a big part of this process. I did not really get the training I think is necessary to handle emotions in this world. My parents were very supportive and available to me. Yet, I believe it is so essential for children to have classes incorporated into their education to help them handle emotions and stress. It could be a class offering very real and tangible tools, tips, and practices to manage the ever-present life experiences that arise—and to let children know that support is available.

When you are not processing, or allowing, what is alive for you, or what you are feeling, it may show up on your skin. This is when a breakout could occur. It has been groundbreaking for me to recognize this tendency.

I encourage you to express and get in touch with any emotions you are feeling. You can do this many ways.

YOU CAN:

- Paint
- Write
- Dance
- Sing
- Talk with a trusted friend who will listen
- Make a collage
- Take a walk

"It is not through thinking that one arrives home: it is through feeling. So, think less, feel more."

— Osho

There are some practices you can do to help feel your emotions.

- One that I have mentioned already and will again because it is such a useful tool is just breathing and being present with what you're feeling. Sitting with the experience, emotion, or challenge and breathing and watching your thoughts and reactions is a simple proactive tool that can help transmute the energy in your body. The key point to feeling your emotions is to be your own observer. Witnessing the feeling, watching its presence, and allowing it to be can give it permission to subside and even dissolve. This is extremely freeing, for it offers relief from doing so much work to try to control or avoid an emotion.

- Find a sense of physical openness within, meaning breath into the emotion, the feeling. It is about being in the physical state of allowing. Here you are welcoming the feeling. When there is little or no resistance in the body physically, you will find total relaxation in the muscles, having let all the tension out of the body. You can just stay in this place and allow the emotion to be and breathe with it. You may want to walk with it, dance with it, or even just sit with it. The feeling at some point may subside. Meditation is a great tool to help the body release and relax. The longer you practice meditation, the easier it will be to enter into this state.

- Accept your feelings. It's likely you are going to feel shame, frustration, anger and embarrassment with chronic skin diseases. What I have discovered is that if you can actually accept these overwhelming feelings, love yourself, and offer yourself deep compassion and forgiveness, then healing begins. When you feel shame around your psoriasis, or frustrated by it, just allow these emotions; even embrace them. Then, send yourself love. By loving and appreciating yourself as any emotion arises, you begin to feel true acceptance. Loving yourself attracts more of the same so we begin to see more love and appreciation in our lives. The Law of Attraction, which states that like attracts like, is at work here. The same goes for our feelings and the circumstances in our lives. If we feel love, even with the tough stuff, then more love shows up.

* Other things that helped me include therapy, the work of Eckhart Tolle, Esther Hicks, Byron Katie, Matt Kahn, and Louise Hay, and many of the books listed in my reference section. Louise Hay's book, *You Can Heal Your Life* is a book that offers lots of affirmations and practices to help you through. Finding people, teachers, authors, friends, family, or anyone or anything that supports and inspires you goes a long way.

Also, it's important to give yourself the time to feel the emotions that arise. Many of us are so busy and do not stop to process or feel what might be upsetting us. It is helpful to allow time for this. Really give yourself space in the moment of an emotional surge to be with it, or if you cannot, designate some time when you can later on that day or even another day. Then, you can just bring up that emotion and sit with it, accept it moving through your body, and stay in an open place.

> *"The allowing of inner states is a
> wonderfully liberating practice."*
>
> —ECKHART TOLLE

WHAT IS ALIVE FOR YOU?

As mentioned earlier, one way to refer to your emotions and what is up for you is by using the word "alive." You can ask a friend what is alive for her or him in regard to any situation. It is a great way to really go deep with someone about a circumstance or situation, and it encourages that person to dive into what is going on for him or her. Many people greet each other by asking how they are; it is a refreshing option to ask some-one what is alive for him or her.

Experiencing emotions, on the whole spectrum of emotions, from sad-ness to joy, is part of life. Each emotion has information for us, and is a wonderful signpost to where we are in the moment and what is alive for us. It can help show us what in our lives we would like to continue focusing on and where in our lives we would like to heal. It is those prolonged feelings of anger and resentment and fear and worry that we ignore, suppress, or avoid that may create restriction in the body and can manifest illness.

"Accept, then act. Whatever the present moment contains,
accept it as if you have chosen it. Always work with it, not
against it. This will miraculously transform your whole life."

— ECKHART TOLLE

3. TAKING RESPONSIBILITY FOR YOUR OWN FEELINGS

"I stopped waiting for the world to give me what
I wanted; I started giving it to myself."

— BYRON KATIE

I wish I had known twenty-three years ago, when I began this journey toward clear skin, that taking responsibility for my own feelings is free-dom. I finally realized this about five years ago when I dove deep into my spiritual/meditation practice, cultivating my connection to the spirit within me. I began by practicing sitting meditation for a period of time, and eventually I began to use affirmations and sit with them for fifteen minutes each morning. The affirmations were powerful words that helped me to find that deep peaceful place. They were words that helped me to contact the source within. I was beginning to see the effects in my life of meditating regularly, yet, to be totally honest, the practice was not initially easy. As I connected more deeply to my spiritual presence, my emotional patterns were revealed quickly and came to the surface. At this time, I had moved to Kauai and am grateful I went through this period in such a pristine setting, paradise on earth.

I uncovered many layers of patterns. For instance, I saw how I was depending on my partner for my happiness. When something arose, I blamed him for how I felt about that situation. He felt pressured and pulled away, understandably. I also recognized that I was insecure and lacked confidence and looked toward him to make me feel good about myself. I thought I was done with this pattern. Not so. This was painful to see but, ultimately, very freeing. There will likely be some patterns you have that will surface for you to see if meditation and connecting to source within becomes part of your daily practice.

I found, and continue to find, peace and happiness within through meditation and following my own inner guidance system. I recognized the freedom and power in connecting to my inner world, and this has been a place to return to continually in my daily life.

During this time, the part of me that was insecure and fearful was uncovered for me to see and witness. I gave my low self-esteem total acceptance, and took steps within and without toward self-empowerment and self-responsibility. For instance, I took flower essences for confidence and jealousy. I would also catch myself almost blaming my partner for something that wasn't his fault and I would just watch myself in this process. I would not take action and say anything. I would take some time for myself and sit with the feeling, instead of react and blame. This has helped me take responsibility for my feelings, and added much ease to our relationship in the process. I continue to practice this and now I do not need to do this often, yet when I do, I notice how quickly I can move through the emotion. I began to see myself grow and spent the next several years deepening my spiritual practice. I was now taking responsibility for my feelings and life, and then--boom. I found opportunity after opportunity to gain true confidence in myself. When I was in massage school, I said yes to a great opportunity; teaching my first class. What happened next was that my healing process began to speed up. Taking responsibility started for me by looking closer at what was ready for me to see. You may have a recurring life pattern or something that is ready for you to witness. Just bring into consciousness what is showing up in your field of reality. Then realize you are able to handle what comes up, and you are in the driver's seat.

The day I began to take responsibility for my life completely is the day that I fully reclaimed my power, after all those years seeking attention from men and finding solace; giving my power away to the men I loved. For me, now, power is about sitting in the knowledge that you are the creator of your world and can take responsibility for your life, your emotions, your relationships, and your story. It is wonderful to stop the blame and feel the strength in knowing no one is responsible for you but you. Ultimately, no matter what someone else chooses to say or do, your reaction or feeling is always yours. Just as you are not responsible for other people's feelings, they are not responsible for yours.

Louise Hayes, in her book *You Can Heal Your Life,* says that disease in the body is often a result of both emotional and thought patterns. She says that psoriasis may be due to a fear of being hurt, deadening the senses of the self, or refusing to accept responsibility for your own feelings. She suggests new thoughts to use as mantras or add into your day: *I am alive to the joy of being. I deserve and accept the very best in life. I love and approve of myself.*

4. Your Feelings Help To Manifest Your Reality

Our emotions help create the circumstances in our life. The reason thoughts are such powerful creators of our experience is that they often conjure emotions that become the precursors to our day-to-day story.

In the past, I spent my life thinking many challenging, negative, and difficult thoughts, which contributed to my psoriasis, other physical challenges, and unpleasant drama in my life. These thoughts created a lot of sadness, anger, fear, and worry within me. Realizing this was a huge piece to the puzzle, though it was definitely not the whole picture.

I was painting a picture in my life based on the feelings I conjured of fear and sadness due to my negative thinking. I was simply used to thinking these thoughts, to allowing them, to feeling these feelings the majority of my time. This helped to perpetuate my life story. When I changed my pattern, my story altered because I decided that feeling good was my number-one priority.

Now, it is important to mention at this point that these emotions—anger, fear, sadness, etc.—are not "bad" or wrong at all. They are great indicators and messengers, and they are inevitable. When these feelings arise, welcome them and allow their presence. Say to yourself, "Oh, there you are, anger! I surely feel you in my body. Oh that is uncomfortable." Be conscious and aware of the feeling's occurrence and breathe with it. Just allow and then watch and when you feel the emotion subside continue on with your day. Then, bring in the emotions of joy and peace when you can. Throughout the day, just think about the actual words joy and peace, and let them come into your energy field. The intention is to accept that anger arises, and consciously create more joy in your life.

Creating a lifestyle that reflects your dreams, your wishes, what you would like to have happen, is part of the fun of life. Begin focusing more on what you want to see showing up in your life. This means not focusing on what you do not want, and it's an integral part of Abraham and Esther Hicks' teaching. Look as often as possible at beauty and anything that brings up positive emotion...whatever that is.

> *"Your observation of the conditions that exist now is*
> *the reason that you keep repeating a pattern that holds*
> *away the things you want. It really is that simple."*

—ABRAHAM-HICKS, SAN FRANCISCO, CA. JULY 19, 2014

How do you begin to look at what you do want, when what you do not want is right in front of you? Well, there are many practices you can incorporate into your life to help you refocus your attention. Refer to the empowerment tools in Chapter 7.

Also, it may help to let go of being angry at others, and yourself, at some point. It may be that it is essential for you to address the person or people involved and speak your truth. This may help to clear some of the anger and resentment. Ask yourself, "How would it feel to let go of that anger and resentment?" Letting go does not mean you need to forget what happened. It does not mean it didn't hurt or that you will be best friends with that person or even have him or her in your life. All "letting go" means is that you can release your hold on the emotion, and the disease that the resentment could be causing you in your body. When you think of that situation or person or event, how does it make you feel? It is probably not a great feeling, and maybe it is time to forgive or begin to think about forgiving. Another thing you could do is write a letter to the person, and let it all out, no inhibitions. It is not necessary to mail the letter. The letter is for you to process and witness yourself.

Often it is yourself that you need to forgive, so start there, if you are ready.

"I forgive myself and set myself free."

—LOUISE HAY

Again, you may not be ready to forgive the person, situation, or yourself. Don't if you are not ready! It is as simple as that.

The empowerment tools that can be found in Chapter 7 can also be used to help with all four of these fundamentals to encourage healing skin.

LIST OF EMOTIONAL CAUSES OF PSORIASIS:

* Lack of self-worth
* Lack of confidence
* Lack of ability to be emotionally self-responsible
* Rigid beliefs
* Shame
* Self-deprecation

YOU CAN BEGIN BUILDING A SENSE OF:

* Worthiness
* Confidence
* Embodiment
* Flexibility
* Contentment
* Self-love

PSORIASIS LOOKS LIKE ANGER

Psoriasis looks irritated, uncomfortable; perhaps like anger would look. It is plaque made up of skin cells multiplying at a very fast rate, replicating out of control. When I was in therapy years ago, my therapist had me draw how I felt about the psoriasis. First, I was timid and not much was expressed, and then I started tapping into my feelings. Wow. I soon learned that I felt frustrated, angry, embarrassed, and scared. I let this out, and it felt so good. Eventually my drawing looked irritated, big, loud, and red. It was interesting to look at. It almost looked like a patch of psoriasis itself.

ALLEVIATE STRESS

Stress comes in many forms--short-term and long-term, acute and chronic, physical and emotional--and can come on suddenly. Many of us deal with stress on a daily basis, as well as long-term. The impact on our bodies can be dramatic and harmful, leading to psoriasis, heart problems, depression, and much more.

My skin showed me there was something off-kilter in my body, something imbalanced physically and emotionally. When I developed psoriasis, I was under a lot of emotional and physical stress, from being bulimic. The stress was causing damage to my intestines and other parts of my body. I stopped being bulimic right before I developed psoriasis. I had also recently quit coffee and cigarettes; this adjustment caused another serious stress for the body.

Emotionally, I was uncomfortable in my skin. I was someone who felt anxiety under a lot of different circumstances. I had a difficult time handling stress and some of the things I did, like smoke cigarettes and drink alcohol, helped me cope. So, when I stopped using unhealthy coping mechanisms, I no longer had any tools or remedies left to handle life. The stress on my body was great. As we have already discussed, lowering stress levels can help your body heal itself quickly and effectively. I suggest using a variety of techniques to alleviate stress. These include daily meditation, breathing techniques, exercise, doing what you love, breathing into the feelings and merging with them, writing, dancing, and drinking relaxing teas such as chamomile and tulsi.

Being in nature is also helpful for reducing stress. Just sitting against a tree, listening to the sounds of the leaves rustling and the birds chirping, or taking a walk can be extremely calming and soothing to the nervous system.

As Dr. Isaac Eliaz suggests, "In clinical studies, we have proven that two hours of nature sounds a day significantly reduces stress hormones up to 800% and activates 500-600 DNA segments known to be responsible for healing and repairing the body."

In the next chapter, I address the spiritual component of clearing skin from within.

CHAPTER 6
Spiritual Healing

* * *

YOU ARE THE CREATOR OF YOUR REALITY

IT IS IMPORTANT TO KNOW that you are the co-creator of your reality. This knowing is the foundation for self-empowerment, and this ultimately can assist in changing your life. If you want to have clear skin and are open to seeing yourself as the co-creator of your life, this can very powerfully support you along the way. The spirit within you is a force that helps you tap into your infinite, powerful self. You do so through meditation and bringing that spirit, that source energy with you throughout your day. So, you and your spirit are like a team, with your spirit reminding you of your innate power.

Direct your energy as often as possible to the beauty of life, even if it is very hard to see and the world around you is filled with challenges. When things seem bleak because you watched the news or you can't pay your bills, this is the greatest time to look for the beauty, to find the joy, to feel your breath and allow the story to just be. Let it be and dive into your body, into what you are feeling. Feel the emotion that is within you, and then, when you're ready, conjure an emotion that would feel better, like calmness or ease or love. Feel that and see what happens.

If you believe that psoriasis is incurable and that you will suffer from it forever, then it may be just that. If you believe that it will be long and hard and difficult to get rid of it, then that may occur.

Now imagine, instead, that you changed your beliefs into know-ing that the psoriasis will go away and it will be easy. If you train your thoughts, what could be called retraining your brain, into this belief, then, again, it can happen. This process of changing your beliefs can take some unraveling. When you've held the same thought for a long time, and then you choose to believe a different thought - one that goes against what most doctors are passing on to their patients - it can be a radical shift. It takes a whole lot of trust—especially in yourself—to change your mind about something. Shifting your thoughts and beliefs, especially around your own health, may call attention to the fact that, as a collective, this culture has placed a whole lot of power into the medical and pharmaceutical realm. This involves shifting your perspective, from one of believing that doctors have all of the answers, to reminding yourself that you actually have immense power within yourself. You have the answer. Here is where the great power of manifestation and miracles lies, as well as a grand knowing that you can change your belief and shift toward allowing what you want into your life. Do you want clear, healthy, vibrant skin? Then start believing this is possible and, even take it a step farther—that clear skin is inevitable. When you can take the steps to believe these new thoughts, you emanate a different vibration, which begins creating changes.

So, where do you focus your attention in your life? Do you tend to look more at the blessings or do you look at the struggles and pain? When you begin to ask yourself these questions, it becomes apparent what you spend most of your time thinking about and why your life is where it is. There is no one else creating your reality besides you and your spirit. So, do not worry. It is totally okay that you are where you are. And, if you want to see something else come into your life, then it may be time to redirect your focus and attention.

This process is a combination of accepting and allowing what is and then redirecting your focus. It has become part of the greatest fun I have in life and in each day. I look forward to seeing how my life will unfold. I wake each morning excited to create more, to feel into what feels good, to watch what shows up from a place of now living a consciously created existence. This practice is pure joy.

I have begun to see all my challenges as opportunities to grow, to empower myself, and to manifest a new, magical, prosperous story. Again, Abraham-Hicks was a great influence for me, especially through the book *Money and The Law of Attraction*. They mention *source energy* very often. I use it when I am, for instance, driving and I feel anxious and impatient. I say to myself, "I am a source energy creator, creating my world." This brings a smile to my face, and I feel a sense of peace. It makes me feel empowered to know that I am walking through this reality, helping to create it.

Here is a simple example of creating your reality. I travel quite a bit to visit my family. Flying for me can be stressful. Growing up, we would fly for vacations, and my dad was very anxious about flying and felt the need to arrive at the airport hours before the flight took off. So now I get a bit anxious, afraid of not making it on time. It is ingrained in me. I am very consciously working to change this pattern so I can stay calm and focused during the journey.

On one particular day I was traveling, and I knew I had a middle seat. I do not like middle seats. They make me feel claustrophobic. There were no other seats available when I booked the flight. So, as I am traveling to the airport, I am thinking thoughts such as...*I just may get an aisle seat. I get to sit comfortably in an aisle seat. I am having a safe journey, smooth and easy.* I literally do not let myself think about the middle seat. I focus on the feelings of ease and joy.

I make it to the gate and ask if there are any aisle seats available and the attendant offers me a seat for fifty-nine dollars, but I don't want to pay this. In my mind, I say, *I still might get an aisle seat*, even though it seems unlikely. I stay open to the possibility of sitting in an aisle seat by thinking positive thoughts and not letting myself think *I will sit in the middle*. I get on the plane in a state of curiosity and wonder, consciously, so as to stay in an energetic place that's open to having what I want happen. I arrive at my seat and notice that there are two large men, one at the window and one at the aisle. I said, pointing to the middle seat, "This is my seat!" The one man responded, "Would you like the aisle seat?"

Grinning, I say, "Definitely." He was traveling with his friend and wanted to sit next to him, which meant him moving to the middle. I was thrilled. This is a perfect example of creating your own reality.

The same thing happened on the way back. I again had a center seat and asked the two nice ladies at the airport if there was an open aisle seat and again they offered a seat with a fee, and I said no. I asked if there were any seats closer to the front, and there was one considerably closer, so I took it. When I got on the plane, nobody was on the aisle seat yet in my row, so I sat in it and waited to see what would happen. A very apologetic man came up and said he was sorry but he was seat 14D, the aisle seat I was in. I moved over and said that was totally okay. Then, a few minutes later he moved to an open window seat a few rows back. This opened up the aisle seat for me. He looked at me and grinned and I grinned back.

The thing is, you cannot control what others do, and you cannot control what they say and choose. But you can control your energy field where you are right now. You can wake up each day and choose to live by peace and kindness and in gratitude as much as you can. It does take some practice, especially if you have been living with depression, anxiety, fear, or post-traumatic stress disorder; if you live in a difficult environment, or if you face any number of other challenges. It is a process. You can begin by allowing yourself to brew up some very positive thoughts. Do this daily, and you may begin to empower your life with what you would like to see unfold.

> *"If you don't rise to the frequency of your own*
> *creation, you cannot realize your own creation."*
>
> —ABRAHAM-HICKS, PORTLAND JUNE 28TH, 2011

RAISE YOUR VIBE...THAT IS YOUR KEY
The most effective tools I have discovered for healing my skin are emotionally and spiritually based. I found that what really took my healing to

the final level and cleared my skin was tuning my vibration to the highest frequency as often as possible. This means tapping into your spirit within and connecting with that part of yourself as often as you can and basically just hanging out there, being there, and letting yourself swim in the presence of the spirit that is alive in you always.

Close your eyes, if you would, for a moment, and take a good easy breath. Place your inner focus on the energy in your body. There may be thoughts that arise. That is okay. Allow them to come up. What I want you to do is pay attention to the alive field of energy within yourself, which can also be called spirit. When you place attention on that, a sense of peace will likely arise. This actually soothes your nervous system immensely and relaxes your muscles, helping to release tension in your body.

You can begin to step out of your focus on your thoughts or your beliefs or even your day-to-day story. Just by placing focus on the spirit within you, you can begin to raise your vibration and lift yourself out of your thought-based reality. This is a practice similar to meditation. In this place, you can feel the difference between focusing on your life's story and the physical reality of your life and focusing on the energy within you. There is a different feeling, one that feels a lot like ease and love.

I look back on my life and realize how much energy I put toward negative thinking and pessimistic thoughts, before I realized how profoundly my life would change if I thought and lived in a more positive way. Waking up to live consciously, meaning choosing what I focus upon and shifting from unconsciously choosing things to consciously making choices each day, has helped me to navigate my own life. When I began to take my power back and navigate my life through thinking uplifting thoughts and feeling joyful and easy, I began raising my frequency. There is an energy field that you are literally emitting and giving off wherever you go and whomever you run into. You are giving off a frequency that is helping you tune into the life that you really want. Just taking time to practice the tools I offer in this book and simply focusing on your inner energy field can change your perception, your vibration, and, hence, the life that you are creating. Now you can see that you can actually create your life knowingly at this point, possibly creating a more peaceful life, and connecting to your spiritual presence.

> *"When you accept that there is a non-physical version*
> *of you, and you embrace it and adore it, and you*
> *practice the frequency of that non-physical part of*
> *you and you allow it to flow into this physical life*
> *experience, then it is a delicious life experience."*

—ABRAHAM-HICKS

SKIN CLEARING

Meditating and focusing on raising my vibration was actually the key to watching the psoriasis fade from my body. As I was focusing on practices to keep me positive and connected to the source within me, my skin completely cleared of psoriasis. I focused each day on the frequency I was emitting, looking to the positive, feeling better, and taking responsibility for my life. And now, every chance I get, and when I remember to do so, I take the opportunity to raise my vibe. When I am standing in a long line at the airport, waiting to get rung up at a store, or on hold on the phone, I use this time to go within and find a place of ease. I have mantras that I say over and over, or I just focus on places in my body where I find tension and consciously release by observing and breathing into that area of tension. This can create massive, quick healing and these potentially mundane experiences become pleasant and even fun.

It was such a blissful delight to see that psoriasis could not live in the physical and spiritual environment I had created for myself. I was allowing myself to feel anything that came up emotionally, yet was continually steering myself back to peaceful, easy feelings. I almost forgot about psoriasis and was just enjoying watching my life unfold in new ways. That is amazing because I had been so focused on the psoriasis for so many years.

Other beautiful things were happening at the same time; my relationship with my partner became really great, and we were enjoying each other immensely and to the fullest, and we were able to handle our challenges with way more ease. I was confident, empowered, and feeling joy more often than before. A brand new sense of being successful emerged from within me. I was fulfilled in knowing that I was creating my reality with the spirit within me. What an empowering world I had just discovered.

I cannot stress to you enough how important creating this new pattern has become in my life. No longer do I find myself dwelling in negative thinking. I have practiced this so much that I have created a new, fresh pattern where I catch myself, again and again, about to go down a road where I am thinking thoughts about how horrible this or that is and how I am not good enough or wise enough or beautiful enough. I see that I am about to spiral out in these thoughts, then I decide that this is not going to do me any kind of good whatsoever, and I choose one of the tools on my rather large tool belt. I eventually conjure up some new, refreshing, nourishing, uplifting, inspiring thoughts, which make for a way more fun and wonderful journey.

This piece of the puzzle is very magical and, at the same time, very real. The way you move through your day and moment and life is very likely synonymous with the health you have. If you are coming from a place predominantly of fear, anger, blame, judgment, or violence, this may create a life attracting similar circumstances, with the same resonance. If you live connected to the spirit within you, in a state of trust and love in your heart at least some of the time, more of this will likely be attracted into it. This is a law of nature, the law of attraction. The book, *The Secret,* along with what many visionaries and spiritual leaders have been teaching for years, describes a very real law of nature. What we think and feel manifests by the law of attraction.

There are many names for the energy alive within you. Here are some: spirit, soul, source energy, divine energy, and God. Whatever you feel comfortable with works; find one that resonates so that you can connect with that alive part within you, and awaken and ignite your connection.

Can you feel what I call source energy within you right now?

Connecting with this every day can give you a real jumpstart on life, even if for just a moment. I choose meditating and talking directly with this field moving through me. It is part of me, this source of energy.

Abraham-Hicks suggests that we raise our vibration to the highest we can as often as possible. This has been, and continues to be, my most often-used tool for experiencing health and empowerment. Raise your frequency so that you have more positive thoughts and feelings. Have positive thoughts and feelings, and you can raise your frequency. It is fun to create thoughts that make you feel amazing. Start with ones that are easy to remember. I am gushing with gratitude toward these teachings; they have helped me live a life I choose to create, no matter what is happening. Quite often I can watch the chaos that may be around me and not get caught up in it at all.

HERE IS MY LIST OF INSTANT FREQUENCY-RAISERS:

* Watching Abraham-Hicks videos on YouTube. This instantly helps me return to peace and a high vibe
* Dancing to my favorite music that inspires me to really let loose
* Breathing deeply
* Listening to certain music
* Taking herbal remedies
* Exercising - even a quick walk will guide me through
* Spending time in nature
* Reciting positive affirmations and really letting them reach my feeling state, so that I feel the emotion deeply
* Looking into someone's eyes
* Getting or giving a massage
* Meditating
* Standing directly on the earth barefoot and breathing
* Taking responsibility for my feelings, my thoughts, and my life
* Connecting deeply with someone

In the next chapter I offer some tools for empowerment.

CHAPTER 7
Tools for Empowerment

* * *

I PUT TOGETHER THESE TOOLS for you to use as a guide or a resource when you need support, are feeling overwhelmed, or are unable to handle circumstances. You may feel off-kilter, frustrated, angry, disconnected, and irritable, and one of these tools may help you shift your vibe, refocus your energy, and/or accept that you feel out of balance or irritable. This is crucial for creating your reality, and helping retrain your brain.

I have mentioned most of these tools throughout the book and they are here in a consolidated list as a reference. They can support you in recreating your experience to the extent that you apply them in your life. They may offer you a chance to have more peace in your daily life. They may also give you a way to implement new ways of being, eating and making choices in your life. There are physical tools, such as herbs and supplements, that I previously mentioned, and then there are these spiritual empowerment tools that may help you tap into your own innate power to live with love and acceptance. It feels so good to just own it, to take charge of your reality.

EMPOWERMENT TOOL #1
INFUSING SELF WITH FEELINGS AND WORDS
This is a great tool to help you raise your frequency and find your way back to a calm, centered state after a challenging emotion or time. It can be used for other circumstances as well.

I have come to base a lot of my personal growth on first feeling the emotions that arise and loving them and then, when the time comes, bringing in feelings such as calmness, joy, and worthiness. It is a balance of the two – accepting the feelings, and then replacing them. It is important to know that we do not want to repress or push away emotions. At the same time we have the choice to redirect our focus.

When I developed psoriasis, not only was my digestive system struggling, but also my nervous system was wired, charged, and in deep need of relaxation and nourishment. A few years ago, I began to infuse myself with emotions and feelings, in the form of words. I was charging myself with peaceful thoughts and emotions similar to charging myself with healthy, nourishing foods, supplements, and herbs. Dwelling on words is a simple and very important tool that you can use anywhere or anytime. I have found much success with doing this on an airplane, on break at work, in the morning when I wake, and many other times. It recharges me, uplifting me to a higher frequency very quickly. It feels so good! I often think of the word *EASE* and then I say to myself ease, ease, ease and feel the resonance of this word surging through my body. This is fulfilling, sweet, and one of my favorite ways to reset my system when it is overwhelmed or I am spinning out of control in a series of unhealthy thoughts. I give major kudos to Esther Hicks, channeling Abraham, for inspiring this very significant practice. They were huge influences for this empowerment tool.

If I am "spinning out," feeling out of control, thinking lots of thoughts that do not feel good, and it is difficult to get out of this state, one thing I do is focus on one word that feels good and breathe with that word as if it was part of me. You can even imagine the word seeping into your body, your tissues, and your cells. Imagine it flowing in there, filling your body with *ease*. If you are feeling stress at work or at home or wherever, find a quiet place and do this. Sometimes, I will even go to the bathroom and lock the door or get in my car if I can't find any privacy. This is an instant vibration shifter.

I take flower essences internally. They are the essences of individual flowers, and they each assist with an emotion or spiritual aspect of life you may be dealing with. For instance, Larch, by Bach Flower Essences, is used for confidence and fear of public speaking. One of my particular daily allies in life, it works on the emotional plane to support me in growth and transformation. Taken regularly, it will help you gain confidence and open up to the potential in yourself. I have been taking flower essences for about fifteen years extremely successfully. I have grown in ways that are profound and have watched the essences help me with very specific patterns and emotions, such as jealousy and despair. So, infusing ourselves with a positive emotion such as ease is like taking a flower essence. Let the emotion simmer in your body and immerse itself into your cells through the word and the feeling, as the flower essence infuses into your body through its liquid potion.

What I also have done is create key words for myself to infuse. When things get rough or I am challenged by what is happening around or within me, after I stop and feel what is alive for me and I am ready to move on, I remember one of the key words, and it helps me to create new thoughts and, hence, create new feelings.

HERE ARE MY MOST OFTEN USED KEY WORDS:

- Worthy
- Opportunity
- Ease
- Love
- Joy
- Happiness
- Kindness
- Peace
- Fun
- Creator
- Empowered
- Jedi

They are the links to finding my way back to peace. This process raises my vibration and sends a message—a signal—out to the universe that I am, say, at ease, open and allowing energy to freely flow through me.

Then, I offer no resistance within myself. Without resistance, the energy of spirit within me—the field of divine love—will freely flow through and to me. This offers me healing on a very deep level, and may offer you peace and a pause in the thought stream you may be accustomed to. It may take you away from your story, and it may be an effective, simple tool for creating healthy patterns of thought within.

You can also use a phrase instead of one word. Just throw an uplifting thought into your stream of thinking that inspires a good feeling. If you are feeling "off" or even if you are just taking a walk, just toss in a thought or two that you like. These fresh thoughts can change the way you feel and can bring positivity to your viewpoint of life. I also love using affirmations to stir up a good feeling.

HERE ARE SOME VALUABLE PHRASES OR AFFIRMATIONS YOU CAN USE:

* I love myself.
* I have vibrant, healthy skin.
* Everything is going to be okay. (This one in particular helps me when the situation is tough or I feel stuck and I need to find my way back to feeling ease.)
* I am grateful for...the sun, music, hip-hop, etc.
* I have immense value.
* I am okay no matter what.
* I made it through that one.

If I feel aggravated or vulnerable about my skin, a practice I do sometimes is to focus with diligent intent on the thought *I have healthy vibrant skin.* I allow this thought to settle within me, and feelings arise like ease, tranquility and joy. I think this new thought regularly, as well as envisioning it, even when my reality is showing me something else. It seemed odd at first to practice this. It was a stark contrast to the feelings I had when I was focusing on the sadness, frustration, and embarrassment. By placing attention on what is possible, on something entirely fresh and new, I began to shift my consciousness around my body and my skin and continued the journey of the scales falling away from my skin.

EMPOWERMENT TOOL #2
EVERYTHING IS AN OPPORTUNITY

This is a powerful tool to change a pattern, redirect your focus, and claim responsibility for your life. You can use it whenever you're inspired to.

This is probably the tool I use most often. Even the toughest of situations can become an opportunity to grow, transform, have compassion, see the best in someone else, and accept and forgive. If you find yourself in a challenging situation, try this; say to yourself, "Wow, this is a great opportunity to…grow, forgive, transform, expand, learn, try something new, help someone, see what isn't working for me, look at something in a new way, practice, empathize, love myself more, accept someone for who they are, see an unhealthy pattern, or choose a new way of doing something." Opportunity is a powerful, transforming word. As soon as I remember to add this word into my thoughts, even for just a moment, my body relaxes, and my perspective on life shifts. Just say the word "opportunity" to yourself when you feel stuck or frustrated about something.

Every challenge is an opportunity! I always resisted my natural inclination to feel what was going on in a room full of people. Being naturally very empathic, I was frustrated that I could feel so much. I resisted this because it scared me, and I did not know how to be this way and not totally take on what others were feeling or going through. I am still developing the skills that enable me not to take on others' feelings and experiences. Staying connected to source is one of these skills. Now, I use this gift of empathy to listen to people's bodies and feelings, and am able to see the immense value in this. Not only am I using this skill to discover what works best for me in terms of feeling, thoughts, and nutrition, I am also helping others find their own power to heal. I have not always seen this as a gift, as it caused me much challenge. I feared it, and I felt overwhelmed with feeling for much of my life. I began seeing that it could be an opportunity for me to tap into my intuitive nature and allow that to guide me through life. Seeing it this way allowed me to let go of the ongoing resistance I had and, hence, embrace my potential.

I now welcome the places in my life that I catch myself resisting, being afraid, having difficult thoughts, or being challenged. I love when I can catch myself in one of these places and see the pattern I have been playing out. As soon as I remember, I look at the opportunity this challenge is offering me. The word "opportunity" has become one of my favorite words to play with. If you see everything as an opportunity, then you are no longer playing victim to your circumstances. You are welcoming what arises as the perfect event or circumstance that you need for furthering yourself. You then claim responsibility for whatever situation you find yourself in. You keep your power; you do not give it away to what arises, or to someone else.

I was in line at Whole Foods the other day, and a woman approached who had a full basket of stuff and placed her basket in front of me in line. I said to her in a nice manner, "Hi, I was next in line." She did not verbally respond but looked at me with a sneer that seemed to express irritation and annoyance. I was merely letting her know I was there. Well, I walked away feeling anger, and then I stopped and realized that, again, this was an opportunity for me to see something in a new way. I began to observe that the subtle situations in life give us a chance to look within ourselves. I realized that lately I, too, have been reacting to subtle exchanges with people with annoyance, and here I could have empathy for her. I never know where someone is coming from without communicating with them. Here was my chance to thank the situation and then move along and play with ways to be less reactive myself. This helped me release the discomfort in my body.

I see life as a playground, and all of the interactions, challenges, blessings, subtleties, and connections become an opportunity to see whom you are, what you have manifested, and how you can grow. It is really about finding the gift in all of it. If someone is unkind to you or another, maybe witnessing this can be a chance to be kinder to yourself and others or help others be more kind. If you are feeling hurt by what someone said, maybe you can remember that this person may only know how to communicate in this way, and that it is nothing personal. Maybe this is an opportunity to let the person know how you feel in a loving, calm manner, offering a chance for a loving exchange and growth for both of you. If you are feeling afraid to address an issue with someone, maybe you can use this as an opportunity to make it fun and joyful by saying to yourself *this will actually be fun.* You could infuse yourself with joy before the talk. It changes our lives dramatically when we can see the situations that arise as little presents for us that give us the opportunity to change our perception and perspective.

EMPOWERMENT TOOL #3
DEEP, DEEP PRESENCE

Tapping into your deep state of presence is a great tool for moving through life with greater ease. Apply this tool anytime, anywhere.

Find yourself immersed in the moment. Close your eyes and feel the fullness of the moment, of what is happening at this point in time. Feel the breeze on your skin, the sun blazing down or the breath in your body, and focus solely on these sensations. Feel the aliveness of your body: your breath, your cells, your muscles, and spirit. Doing so can bring much ease and support you in letting go of the constant stream of thoughts. It encourages a calm feeling to emerge; you may release all the tension in your body and just appreciate the feeling of being alive. It is like putting a magnifying glass on the present moment. Then, allow yourself to touch and meet the spirit within. Feel its presence. Feel it to the fullest. Relax into it with your body by letting go of any tensions, stresses, concerns, or anything you are holding onto. Bask in this. It can be a glorious feeling. Be with it, dance with it, and walk with it as long and as much as possible.

I bring this presence with me as often as I can remember when I go to work, go out to dinner, and give a massage or a health consultation. It brings a peaceful, loving energy to the situation you are in. I have been told my energy is very calming, and I absolutely love this. I attribute this to the connection I focus on within myself in the presence of the moment. Bringing your presence into a situation with another is a blessing for them because it offers this connection to them and will allow spirit in. This is all I could ever ask for - to help others remember to be serene. It is such a gift for that person. Eckhart Tolle inspired me in his book, *Through the Open Door*, in which he reminds us that we walk as a blessing when we are bringing this deep state of presence into any situation or with any person. It offers a calming, tranquil energy.

Another exercise you can add into your practice is to visualize the cells within you. Imagine one particular cell and see it in your mind's eye. Then, imagine the center of the cell and see and know that it goes on infinitely in the center. You can envision this at any time and it brings you to a place of tapping into the deep spaciousness that you are.

We are made of the stars, the earth, and space. So, literally, the cells that reside within have no ending. Nassim Haramein discusses this in his work and research in the field of unified physics, which looks at the inter-connectedness of all things and nature, and is shown in his Resonance Project. He says that as far as the sky and universe extend beyond us, so each cell goes within us. There is a universe within each cell. WOW! Okay, so that is a big thought. Knowing this quite delicious bit of information is an incredible tool that helps us to always remember that we have an infinite source of energy to tap into and exude. In doing so, we have a vibrational field that we take with us, wherever we go, with every breath we take.

There is such peace that lies in that full experience. This is what I see as the "kingdom of heaven," that Jesus refers to. To me, this is the place where we can find pure heaven on earth. We can feel the incredible joy of being here, right now, experiencing the connection to the depths of our soul.

EMPOWERMENT TOOL #4
REPATTERNING

Repatterning – changing a pattern that you've been repeating for a long time - can be a big contributor to clearing skin. You can change any pattern you like.

HERE ARE THREE WAYS REPATTERNING CAN BE ACCOMPLISHED:

1. By continually doing something differently, therefore creating a fresh way of moving through life.

   For example, I notice that my mind is about to think some thoughts that will most likely feel icky. I can tell I am about to take that road and I nip it in the bud. I find that feeling that I go to every day when I meditate, when I look to source, the feeling I feel when I am relaxed, when there are no tightened muscles, when I am looking to the place within that is infinite. Then I just look towards that and choose that option, instead of the option of continuing to focus on the thought that makes me feel sad, depressed, or awful. I look to that place within that is peace to me, a place where love resides and where I am deeply connected. You could say there is a muscle that has been strengthened, a muscle of connection to peace and love, or, simply said, a muscle of connection. The more I go there, the easier it is to choose going there. The more I go there, the stronger my muscle of connection becomes. This is repatterning.

   It may take some practice to get to this point where you can stop yourself from spiraling out in thought. It also may take practice to find that feeling place of peace with ease. For me, it has become such a common feeling that I can elicit it just by acknowledging it. I have trained myself into becoming a "Jedi", as it were, focusing on the calm within the storm and maintaining focus there. This builds inner strength and trust in your own power, and is very important to creating your own world because it gives you confidence and an excitement that you do have control in your life. It's a relief and changes the whole game. I use the word "Jedi" to remind me to go within and look to the beautiful, strong place I have within myself.

   You see, you are very used to doing something a certain way, so it is easy to continue to return to that way of doing it. Yet, when you decide to do something totally different, you begin to create a new way of handing a situation.

Here is an example: I had eczema on my hands for a period of time, and it was painfully itchy. I would just scratch it and scratch it, and then I would be in more pain. I remember once I was in so much discomfort I started to cry, and my dear friend was there to help me see that there is another way of handling it. She gave me some ice. She told me that I was deep in this pattern of having an outbreak of eczema, scratching it, it getting worse, and then it hurting. Immediately I began creating a new pattern. I began using ice to ease the itch and pain instead of scratching. I would also look to my muscle of connection, as mentioned above. It took me continually choosing this to begin to change my pattern. Now, I do not itch very often and, when I catch myself scratching, I return to new ways of handling it. This is one example of repatterning.

2. Repatterning can be accomplished by focusing on what beliefs resonate with you, and what beliefs are the basis for creating and manifesting your life. So, think about it. If I believed what my skin doctor believed, that I would have psoriasis forever and that it is incurable, then I would live by this premise. I would think this thought regularly, and the result would likely show up for me in my life. When I decided that anything is possible and I can heal my own body, then I set forth a whole different tone to live by. After many years of giving away my power to beliefs I picked up from others, such as doctors or my friends or parents, I decided it was time to let my own power shine. I began by allowing in the thoughts that would support me on my journey toward health. I knew thinking that psoriasis was incurable would not work. So what would I have to lose to think the thought, *psoriasis is curable*?

3. Just by being your own observer, you can change a pattern. I had a lot to witness inside myself; patterns to look at and to love and accept.

"Every time you discover a mind pattern, an old mind pattern acting itself out, a self-image, defensiveness, grasping, clinging, the moment you become aware of patterns, the awareness or the knowing is not part of that. That's why it's so wonderful. The more you discover that's unconscious in you, the better."

—ECKHART TOLLE

My whole being unraveled, meaning that the patterns that were holding this "dis-ease" in place were seen, brought to the forefront, so I could be aware of what was creating my world and let it go. Bringing things to the forefront is letting what comes up be seen, consciously, instead of it unconsciously existing in your life. What comes up may be an emotion, a reaction; you're noticing how you are handling situations in your life. It is observing with a different eye, as you see yourself move through your days. Watch yourself, and what you say and feel. If, for instance, you scratch your skin a lot, why don't you simply observe yourself next time you feel compelled to scratch? See what is up for you; your feelings, your physical reactions, your jaw, and your breath. How do you feel? Notice the emotions and sit with them. Feel into it and breathe with it. When my patterns were brought to the forefront, I initially found it very difficult to witness. I saw that I was very insecure and lacked confidence in myself. I saw that I was grasping, reaching for anything to give me security and stability, and I knew as I witnessed this that I was ready to look to myself instead of others. I began to observe my life, to watch how I was acting and feeling, and this helped lessen my emotional pain. Then I could choose to rebuild my patterns, lovingly, gently, and deliberately. This was a process and did not happen instantly, but repatterning sure did hasten the skin clearing.

As I work on repatterning, I do my best to accept what comes up, no matter how awful the thought or feeling is. Then, I allow it to just be. I do not forcefully repress or deny it. I just allow it, and then I redirect my focus. It is like *The Wizard of Oz*...just follow the yellow brick road. There are a lot of roads to choose from. I choose the road that leads to my own power as often as I possibly can.

EMPOWERMENT TOOL #5
VISUALIZATIONS

Visualizing clear skin regularly has been a helpful tool for me in clearing my skin. Visualizations can be used in any area of your life.

When I first began visualizing clear skin on my not-so-very-clear skin, it was very difficult for me. I was so focused, in my day-to-day life, on the fact that I had psoriasis and the concept that it was ugly and hideous. I held trauma around this subject. I was always concerned that people could see it and wondered what they would say about it. I was sure I was being judged and that I was grossing people out. I really felt like a monster. So, it was difficult for me to see it gone when, for so long, all I could see was its presence. I had been feeling so many uncomfortable feelings; it was hard to conjure positive ones around my skin.

I started visualizing myself before I developed psoriasis. I had a memory of myself in a bathing suit with clear skin at around age fourteen, and I would visualize myself at that time, with clear skin. I would remember how that felt; like ease and joy. This was my visual reference, and each time I practiced this visualization, it became easier and easier. Eventually, I could imagine my skin clear in the present.

With the continued practice of visualization, I created a new situation in my life, a new pattern. Eventually, I became used to seeing this visual and also feeling what it brought up, and this helped support me in finding serenity in my life. Frustration was more common up until I started meditating and visualizing. Now, peace has become a dominant feeling in my life and one that I continue to return to.

I do a regular visualization when I am in sitting meditation: I see myself with clear skin all over my body. Yours could be a visual of you from the past or one in the present. The vision is crucial to this process. See it and then feel what it feels like to have clear skin, to feel your knees, your elbows, your scalp, wherever psoriasis is, totally free of psoriasis. Embody clear skin. This is essential. What does this feel like? Relief and contentment will probably be feelings you experience. Let those feelings in. For me, I sink into the feeling that comes up, allow it to really settle in, and continue to meditate on the feeling as long as possible, and I keep returning to it. I take note of this sensation in my body and conjure it up going forward when I remember to do so. I do this when I am in line at the bank or in traffic, or I simply add it into my meditation practice. Basically, it is a great practice to do whenever you feel inspired. As I do this visualization, the tension in my body begins to dissolve.

EMPOWERMENT TOOL # 6
LISTENING

Listening to the spirit within is a great tool to develop to help guide you on your path towards clear skin.

It is a skill I have been practicing for years now. It involves tuning your senses to the deep place inside and listening from that place instead of from your thoughts and what you see going on around you. You go within to that place inside that is still, yet also speaking to you, and look to this for guidance on your path.

There is a way to listen without hearing words. This is listening to your feelings and sensing from a place of intuition. A place that is deep in your body, beyond your body, will communicate with you; it is your spirit, which is always dwelling in and about you. When you look toward this, you can listen with your heart, your inner eye, your feeling body, or simply your ears. You begin to open up to the spaciousness within, where true magic can activate divine guidance.

You can stop what you're doing and pay attention to this voice, this feeling that arises within you, that may be leading you to your most joyous path. It can come in many forms: a voice, a feeling, a vibrational hum, a knowing, or some other way that is unique to you. You can begin to pay attention to the subtleties going on within your body. The voice is different from the one that comes from your emotional body; from fear, anger, joy, or sadness. This voice may come at times when you are charged with emotional energy. The voice I am referring to is your soul voice.

It is guiding you, based upon the questions, visions, wishes, and dreams you have and the energy you are emitting. The questions you can ask it are those that you ask the universe or the spirit residing within or whatever you pray to. It might be the questions you write in your journal. If your focus is to clear your skin, then you will likely be led in that direction. There is groundbreaking information to resurrect from the depths within. You may not even realize it when it is happening. We are powerful creators, continually creating the world around us from the world within us.

Here is one way that you can hone this skill. You can listen completely and fully with deep presence to others. Listening deeply to others involves listening to someone without distraction. You just sit and focus on them, their words and their energy and listen. At the same time, you can take soft, deep breaths and tap into your own energy, instead of your mind thinking. Practicing listening to others in this way can really help you get better at listening from within.

EMPOWERMENT TOOL #7
FOCUSING ON THE GOOD

In adding this daily practice into my life, I have watched the unfolding of a more serene life for me.

I love this tool. It is so beautiful to look at someone, no matter who they are, and see their best. You have a chance to notice their best qualities and see beyond their story, fears, insecurities, reactions, and anger. To really look at someone without any judgment and fully accept that person as they are is a massive gift to that person and yourself. You are free then from assumptions and expectations. It is extremely liberating to just allow that person to be. Everyone has divine energy flowing through him or her. What if you could see that in your mom, your doctor, your lover, and even the most challenging person in your life? What is beautiful about them? Let them shine. See them shine.

This practice offers the other person a gift - a dose of unconditional love and acceptance. You are seeing that person through the eyes of non-judgment. When someone sees the best in you, it truly feels wonderful. You are not asked to be anything more or less than you are. This is freedom.

You can also focus on the good in your life regularly and as often as you can. This is a great practice to do every day. It is fun, and once you get the hang of it, it can be easy too. Even if everything looks bleak and feels challenging and not so good, you can begin to just let it be. Then, choose something great in your life. It could be the delicious lunch you made or that your room is clean or your bed is cozy. It may be that you love your dog. Just dwell on that.

I am grateful for something every day, no matter what. I am grateful to be alive, cruising around in a body and seeing the story get better and better.

"You walk as a blessing on this earth."

—ECKHART TOLLE

EMPOWERMENT TOOL #8
SELF-OBSERVATION

Self-observation is a tool to use daily to help shift patterns in your life. It can be used at any time to help in many circumstances.

Being the observer of the circumstances, feelings and thoughts that you have is very different from letting the circumstances, feelings and thoughts take over your reality. When you watch what is happening, you can make a choice to see what is alive for you instead of become what is alive for you.

Having skin challenges helped me clear up my inner game. It helped me to see that there is an opportunity to release negativity by seeing where my thoughts go when I am focusing on a skin breakout, and where they go in general.

One way to feel into this is by sitting still in a quiet, peaceful space where you know you won't be interrupted, closing your eyes and watching your breath inhale and exhale. Begin to see yourself from within. This is perfect if there is any discomfort anywhere in your body. See how you may be holding something in your physical body. It may show up as a tight muscle, for example your jaw or shoulder muscles. Are you clenching your teeth? Watch and see what your body is up to. Then, when you think a thought, feel whatever comes up in your body. Do you react in any particular way? Do you twitch or tighten your muscles? What do you feel? Do you feel sadness, as if you may cry, or frustrations, as if you want to scream? Does your psoriasis itch or is there any other issue that is causing pain? Just allow it, let it be and watch yourself. Watch your feelings and your body and see what comes up. It may be a little uncomfortable. It may not.

This may help you change your patterns by bringing your awareness into daily situations, to what you think, feel, and do. You can take this tool with you everywhere. Put direct attention on the discomfort. Look at it. Feel it. Yet, stay with it. What you are doing is putting space around the challenge, letting it just be. There is no fighting or resisting it in this moment. This practice may help reset the pattern which wants to resist. There is no need to do anything but observe. Be with this, and it may be that, just by watching and not judging or doing anything, you may start to feel calm and centered.

I often have a tight jaw when I think harsh thoughts about myself. It sends me a message that I am spiraling into a negative thought pattern when my jaw is clenched. I scratch my skin when I feel anxious and fearful and am thinking thoughts that feel uncomfortable. So, when I catch myself scratching, I can almost always match it with a challenging thought or emotion. Then I take a deep breath, stop any activity I am doing, if I can, and just watch and observe. I stay in deep openness and observation. The pain will usually transform. The more you can watch what comes up non-judgmentally, the more you are shifting the pattern.

In Chapter 8, I discuss the joys of being free of psoriasis and outline the steps I took in clearing my skin.

CHAPTER 8
Free of Psoriasis

✳ ✳ ✳

ONE DAY, I LOOKED DOWN at my knees and elbows and realized that the psoriasis was no longer there. This is literally what happened. After all those years of shame and anger at my body, I was now free from the constant presence of psoriasis. I felt joy, praise, and gratitude for having come to that place of accomplishment and deep satisfaction. All those years of focus and determination had paid off. For twenty-three years, I had very thick plaque covering me; and then it was gone. I was, and frankly still am, elated. I am thankful, so thankful for my commitment and for the journey that gave me the gifts of an elevated vibration and an intimate relationship with myself and the spirit within me.

What I realize now is that I found the peace and confidence within myself *first* and then the psoriasis faded completely. I needed to know my self-worth deeply before it disappeared from my skin. Our bodies are perfect. They are true mirrors for what is alive within us emotionally. People often have the thought and, hence, the belief, that they need to have something happen in the physical world before they find peace, healing, love or joy. For instance, someone who has psoriasis may desperately want their psoriasis to fade away so they can then find confidence and peace. What I learned is that I needed to find the peace and confidence without it being gone. Then, it was gone.

Here's the big lesson for me, the biggest lesson of all: We are more powerful than we think. We are really creators of our own reality.

The first doctor I saw told me I would have psoriasis for the rest of my life. I was terrified and devastated by that, and filled with sadness and shame to think that I had no control over my own body and that I would have these patches of scales forever. But I guess that doctor was wrong, because it has been gone for over two years now, and I know that I helped clear it. I am clear that I do have control over what happens to my body. Initially, I felt helpless and that I was doomed to have this skin disease indefinitely. In the moment this trauma occurred, there was no way for me to see that this was actually exactly what I needed to wake up and to become more responsible and spiritual. Without having the tools then that I have developed now, I was not able to see that this event was actually a wonderful opportunity for me to transform my life. Now I see that it was, hands down, the best thing that could have happened to me.

I had to start seeing where I was giving my power over to others, how I was choosing beliefs according to other people's ideas, not mine. When I was a kid, I used to see the news on the TV in my parents' room, and it seemed so silly to me. I questioned the validity of what I was watching. Later I remembered this part of me, the part that questions what doesn't feel good to me, what doesn't seem true. Esther Hicks and Abraham say, "A belief is a thought we keep thinking." (*The Vortex* CD, Track Nine.) A belief is a thought, and who is to say that just because someone thought it enough to create a belief around it, we should listen to it and abide by it?

So I woke up to psoriasis disappearing from my reality, and I now believe that in choosing to believe something, anything, such as psoriasis is incurable, we are actually likely manifesting that belief. As soon as I really knew, deep in my body, that I am powerful, then the psoriasis was gone. Then I knew I was the one helping make my reality happen. These eyes, these thoughts, these feelings, are so potent that they assist in manifesting the life I am living now. Each day, you emit an energy field as you move through the world. This field attracts to it more of the same. So, wouldn't it be a good idea to start watching what we are putting out there? Hell yes!

Wake-Up Call

Whether you just developed psoriasis or have had it for a few years or your entire life, it could be your wake-up call to your potential. Health issues are often, if not always, a message that something needs to be seen or heard, that there is something that would really benefit from a change. For instance, one's lifestyle may need shifting in order to allow the body to find a clear path toward health and balance again. Health challenges may also occur because your body and soul are calling out for love. I now see psoriasis as a gift, a real treasure in opening my eyes and heart to a very conscious, inspired life that I would not have embarked on without this incentive.

One day, I realized that I needed to take responsibility for my life and learn to make healthy choices. I started down a very different path than I had ever been on, and I have spent the last twenty-plus years on a health quest, discovering what I need to do to allow my body to thrive. I gained much knowledge, information, and insight that I hope can help assist you along the way.

My time and effort have paid off, and all of the hiding and shame are behind me now. Those days are gone. In fact, I am so proud and happy of my skin, I often wear "booty shorts" and very short skirts: it's as if I am making up for the hermit years, when I was hiding my skin from the world. Some folks have thought I was crazy to wear those revealing outfits, but I don't care a bit! It feels like freedom.

Even better than the feeling of freedom that comes from finally having clear skin, I have found true connection, the best "high" ever, the truest living I have ever experienced. It is the connection to the deep place within myself, the place where I meet God, where there is eternal ongoing peace and bliss. That is how I healed my body, and it is available to everyone.

Praising Psoriasis

Psoriasis. Thank you for helping me to find the beauty within myself, for me to see that I have a very strong will and a vivacious spirit, ready to enjoy and embrace life. Thank you for waking me up to the knowledge that I have a whole world inside myself.

Thank you for helping me see where I need to grow, where I have places to transform, and where there are cobwebs that need cleaning.

I gave a whole lot of time and energy to clearing you, to wishing you away, and I am grateful for learning to trust--to trust that, no matter what, I was okay. I actually learned to love you, to accept you, because you were a part of me. No matter what was on my skin, no matter what other people thought of me, no matter what even I thought of me, I was always fine.

Psoriasis, I give thanks for how you have refined my taste, so that I love the taste of simple foods. I thank you for showing me that the deliciousness in food comes from how naturally it is grown. I love fresh avocados from the tree, wild nettle juice, lemon and water, sautéed veggies in coconut oil and sea salt. These simple creations are delicious to me and help me to thrive. There was a time when eating a pizza with everything on it and cheese fries and a Philly cheese steak would be the only thing that would satiate me. That feels like a lifetime ago. Psoriasis, you helped me transform my lifestyle so that I could appreciate a true holistic way of life, one where I listen to my inner voice showing me the way, where I follow this guidance, and where I trust that I will be satisfied and nourished.

I give thanks for having this disease. Without it, I would not be so attuned to my body and spirit's needs. I would not be so vibrant, and feeling so much authentic gratitude each and every day of my life.

I give thanks that the skin on my knees, elbows, and hips is now smooth, soft skin. The skin on my face used to be rough, dry, and often blotchy with redness, eczema, and acne, even just a few years ago. Now, my skin is softer than it has been since I've been an adult. At times, I find myself grinning from ear to ear when I feel my skin. This has been a dream of mine for my whole life. Being someone who always had skin problems from my teenage years on, it is a blessing. I love the way I look in my forties--way better than I did in my twenties and thirties.

I also give thanks for being able to pass on this information to you, my readers, so that you can see the blessing that you have been given by psoriasis, whatever that may be for you. It may be that having psoriasis will help you to love yourself and deepen your relationship to yourself and the spirit within you. Maybe this information will be a guide to give you inspiration and support and see that there is a possibility for peace and clear skin.

I spent twenty-three years studying, researching and experimenting on my self and I am thankful that because of this you don't have to do a lot of research yourself. *Psoriasis Free and Clear* contains all the information I gained so you have a resource of information to help you along your way.

Mine has been a very long path of self-discovery. I let go of many aspects of myself that were no longer helping me in any way in my life, and this opened a path of continual expansion and evolution. When I began this journey, I was scattered, self-loathing, and living with depression and low self-esteem. I now spend most of my days feeling centered, content and healthy.

So, today, I give thanks for psoriasis, for the journey it took me on, and for its help in uncovering my highest potential to live in this life.

When things get a little tough or I forget how powerful I am, I look at my knees and elbows. I remember that I have played a huge part in clearing my skin. I have found the way of peace, and this means more to me than anything, even more than having clear skin.

YOUR UNIQUE PROCESS

Certain people tend toward lung problems, digestive problems or urinary tract issues. Others tend to have skin problems. Those who tend to break out on their skin in some form, when out of balance, under stress, or overwhelmed, will feel reassured that there are ways to support yourself during the process so it is easier to move through. I am here to let you know that tapping into what your body is telling you, along with accepting it and also loving yourself, can make a massive difference in your body's response. It is possible that having psoriasis is actually helping you find your way to wellbeing.

Clearing your skin will ultimately be your own unique journey. I offer this guide as a resource to refer to and gain support along your way and to help you begin to implement some or many of the tools here. I want to help expedite your journey and help you see all the angles you can play with. I like to use the word "play", instead of "work", as much as possible, so it becomes more fun, light, and easy to embark on this road. Commitment, change, and presence can be actually enjoyable. This I can attest to. It is sometimes uncomfortable, yet this does not last too long when you focus on the good in your world as much as possible.

This book is a download of key information that can help you to welcome in a healthier lifestyle that meets your particular needs and wants, and allows you to express your highest self. Your sovereignty can take you beyond other people's beliefs. You can also practice some new, fresh ways of seeing what is currently in your field of reality. Clearing my skin has been an incentive for me every single day to develop a strong will. It does take commitment, and if you are up for this commitment, then you may be on your way to your heart's desire.

I Am Successful

I spent most of my life thinking that I did not have a focus. I did not have children. I am not married. I did not have a job I loved (until now). I have watched many people in my life have a primal focus for work that they put energy, dedication, and belief into year after year. I struggled with finding something that I truly loved, something that I too could focus on. Then, I woke to the realization that healing my body has been my life's "work." Many people may not recognize my accomplishments, and that is okay. They may see that I have a very unique lifestyle and have chosen to live very differently than most. I see myself as a woman who has accomplished much and is successful in my own way. I choose to live a life with a strong emphasis on self-healing, on finding what it will take for me to thrive at my highest. Then, I can pass on this information to others and truly help them. To me, sharing this information is the greatest gift.

What I want to get across here is that your valuing yourself is crucial to your empowerment and embodiment. If you want to be in your body, feel happy, and create the life you want, look at the positive elements in your life. See yourself as the prosperous being that you are, even if you have until now seen yourself as not enough, as not successful, not beautiful, not this or that. See if you can shift that perspective; it will change your life.

I accomplished success by healing my physical body. I used to struggle with the thought *I am not successful*, and this really caused me a lot of suffering, to the point of depression. Now, I see that I am indeed successful. I stuck with this path to empowering myself for many years. I regained my power through this journey and, for this reason, I feel completely fulfilled. When I start getting down about the insanity that I witness or feel in this world, I very often remember the personal love I have found for myself, and allow myself to feel the fullness of its accomplishment.

SUMMARY OF THE STEPS I TOOK IN CLEARING PSORIASIS

I want to lay this out in a way that gives you very clear information about the steps to take for your skin's clearing:

1. Eliminate any foods and drinks that are aggravating you.
2. Add delicious, nutritious foods to your diet, along with nourishing drinks that work for you.
3. Start taking supplements that support you in thriving.
4. Create lifestyle habits that nourish you.
5. Address emotions with these four fundamental steps:
   * Develop a genuine, deep love for yourself.
   * Allow yourself to fully feel your emotions.
   * Take responsibility for your feelings.
   * Know that your feelings help to manifest your reality.

6. Have tools and practices to refer to that can help you continually return to a high frequency, deal with the challenges of your day, find self-love and empowerment, help create the life you want, and have more peace in your life.

THESE INCLUDE EIGHT EMPOWERMENT TOOLS:

* Infusing self with feelings and words
* Everything is an opportunity
* Deep, deep presence
* Repatterning
* Visualizations
* Listening
* Focusing on the good
* Self-observation

You can choose to take a journey now into finding your way to your healthiest self, the most amazing version of you. Psoriasis may have showed up in your life as a doorway to changing your lifestyle in a way that will bring you into a vibrant way of being. It may be there to help you reevaluate your choices and find the ones that best nourish you.

I am not asking you to implement all of my suggestions and change your whole life. I am asking you to take a look at where you are now, create an image of what you would like to see, and allow the rest to fall in place. Let it fall in place. See what you want to manifest. Do you want to eat differently? Do you want to feel peace with where you are now? What steps can you take to create more peace in your body? What is it that you want to create? Right now, you may want to have clear skin, free of psoriasis. No matter what it is you want to create, you are the holder of the key to your happiness. Now that's a fun belief to play with!

If you are feeling overwhelmed, or you are ready to get serious about improving your psoriasis naturally, I am available to do nutritional and empowerment consultations to help you find the right individualized herbs, supplements, foods, and practices to help you thrive. You can contact me at www.SkinSoulutions.com or mjberkman@yahoo.com.

Now, I offer some recipes to prepare for skin clearing.

CHAPTER 9

Recipes for Skin Clearing

∗ ∗ ∗

I CREATE RECIPES THAT ARE simple, delicious, and very nutritious. This is what I love to do, and it has become my hobby and a joy in my life. I have had so many health issues through the years. As I gained knowledge and information on what would be the optimum foods for me to eat, I began playing with recipes that I would enjoy and that would be great for my skin and health. I then created a bunch of simple recipes that are my staples the majority of the time. These recipes have been a very large part of my life for many years now and have been a basis for helping to clear my skin.

THE CRITERIA FOR MY RECIPES ARE AS FOLLOWS:

- Use organic ingredients as much as possible, except if you are in a pinch or unable to get any.
- Use around eight ingredients or less in each dish.
- Use coconut and olive oil, and stay away from hydrogenated oils that are difficult to digest when cooked at high temperatures. Their structure is altered in such a way that it becomes like a foreign substance to our body.
- Use low-glycemic sweeteners, such as xylitol and coconut sugar. Use raw honey, which has a higher glycemic index but enough nutritional value that I still recommend using it.
- Eat only wild-caught fish and 100% grass-fed meat.
- Be in a good mind space when preparing meals. If not, wait to prepare food or do a simple energy clearing before beginning.

You can say to yourself, "I let go of anything through the day causing tension and I call in divine energy to move through me while I prepare food". At the same time, you can visualize the release of tension, and divine energy flowing through you.

* Check in and make sure you feel aligned and at peace with what you are choosing to put in your body.

Marjy's Recipes

Breakfast Ideas:

CHIA CEREAL
Serves: 1
⅓ c. chia seed
½ c. hemp seed
3 tbsp. xylitol
A healthy pinch of sea salt
A healthy handful of cacao nibs
A healthy handful of fresh fruit – bananas, blueberries, strawberries, or other fruit
A healthy handful of whatever organic nuts or seeds you desire, raw, sprouted or roasted plain or in just sea salt
¾ c. water

Soak chia in water for 20 minutes. Stir periodically. Add the rest of the ingredients and serve; I love it with sliced apples.

Chia can solidify your stools and bring regularity. You do not need to eat a lot for this result. A little bit goes a long way.

DELISH FISH
Serves: 1
1 piece wild-caught fish
½ tsp. coconut oil
⅛ tsp. sea salt
Squeeze of lemon juice
Sprig of dried herb such as rosemary or thyme, or a dried spice blend to cover one side of fish, such as garam masala or ginger.

Add lemon, salt, and herbs or spices to fish and then sauté in coconut oil heated to medium temperature for 3 minutes. Flip and cook 2 more minutes. Remove from pan and put on a baking dish in a preheated oven at 300° for about 5 more minutes. The amount of time you cook the fish depends on the thickness of the fish, the type of fish, and how rare you want it.

Fish is an easy-to-digest form of protein, and I find it a nice breakfast food. It gives me sustained energy throughout the day.

PROTEIN POWER BAR
Serves: 2
3 tbsp. almond butter
1 tsp. hemp powder
2 tsp. xylitol (from birch)
⅛ tsp. sea salt
A healthy handful of cacao nibs
1 tsp. ground chia seed
1 small handful goji berries or mulberries

Mix all of the ingredients in a bowl. Press into ball shapes and keep in freezer.

This is great for breakfast, hiking, before or after working out, air travel, or anytime you want some condensed, yummy, nutritious food. It is high in protein, magnesium, fiber, and essential fatty acids. Some of the bars that you can purchase, even at natural grocery stores, are very high in sugar and also tend to have things added to them unnecessarily. It is nice to have something like this that is very high in nutrients and fulfills the need for something replenishing and hearty.

LUNCH IDEAS:

WILD SALMON SALAD

Serves: 1
1 piece (cooked) or 1 can wild-caught salmon
1 tsp. sea salt
½ large avocado
Pinch of black pepper
Juice from half of a lemon

Mash all ingredients together into a salad. When squeezing in the lemon, you can take out the seeds first or use a lemon squeezer. I like this dish with lots of lemon and salt.

The omega-3 fatty acids in wild salmon are high. Taking fatty acids internally helps soften the skin from the inside. Wild salmon is anti-inflammatory and rich in many nutrients, such as vitamins E, B12, D, and selenium.

VIBRANT SKIN SALAD

Serves: 2
3 c. green cabbage (finely sliced)
2 tbsp. olive oil
2 tsp. apple cider vinegar
¼ tsp. sea salt
2 tbsp. hemp seed

Put cabbage in a bowl and add all of the other ingredients. Massage the ingredients together. This is a delicious, simple salad that is great for your skin and created in just a few minutes.

Green cabbage is a food that has really helped me with my skin. It is a "go-to" food when I want to clear up acne. I notice that after I eat a cabbage salad, my skin looks better than it did before. It is rich in vitamins C and A and beta-carotene and, if it's raw, sulfur. These nutrients all help with the health and vibrancy of the skin. It is high in amino acids that help fight inflammation.

PUMPKIN SEED DIP
Serves: 3
1 c. pumpkin seeds, soaked
1 tbsp. coconut oil
1 tsp. olive oil
¼ tsp. sea salt
¾ tsp. Ume plum paste
½ tsp. kelp powder
¾ c. water

Strain and rinse the pumpkin seeds after soaking for 4 hours. Blend all ingredients together in Vitamix or food processor. Put a scoop on a salad or use it as a dip for sliced veggies.

Pumpkin seeds are very high in zinc, a nutrient that's essential for healthy skin and for boosting the immune system, and that has been known to help heal acne.

BUTTERNUT CREAM
Serves: 2
3 c. chopped butternut squash
2 tsp. coconut oil
¾ tsp. sea salt
2 c. broccoli
1½ tbsp. sage

Chop veggies and steam with the chopped sage for about ten minutes. Put in a high-powered blender with the rest of the ingredients and blend to a creamy, delicious soup.

In general, blended foods are great for those with compromised digestion and an excellent option for people who want to easily assimilate their food and may be having a hard time doing so. The butternut squash has lots of beta-carotene, and vitamins A and C, which are all beneficial to the health of the skin.

DINNER IDEAS:

HEARTY HAMBURGER
Serves: 1
¼ lb. 100 % grass-fed meat of choice (beef, buffalo)
1 tsp. coconut oil
Pinch of sea salt
Juice from half of a lemon

Make meat into burger. Heat coconut oil on medium and cook burger with salt and lemon for about 3 minutes on one side, then flip. Cook to taste.

I love to give thanks to the animal for its food and medicine before I eat. I close my eyes, place my hands around the meal, and express gratitude toward the food.

SUPER SIMPLE SALAD
Serves: 1
1 c. chopped greens of choice (romaine, red leaf, arugula)
1 sliced cucumber and/or red pepper
2 tbsp. olive oil
1 tsp. apple cider vinegar (or lemon juice)
1 handful of pine nuts
¼ tsp. sea salt
$1/8$ tsp. raw honey

Mix olive oil, apple cider vinegar (or lemon juice), pine nuts, sea salt, and honey together in a bowl. Add to remaining ingredients.

Eating some greens with meat will bring balance to the meal. The meat on its own is acidic, so the addition of greens provides sufficient alkalinizing properties to harmonize the meal.

SUPER SAUTÉ

Serves: 1 or 2

One bunch greens of choice (kale, collards, mustard greens, or whatever is local and fresh)

2 tsp. coconut oil

½ tsp. sea salt

1 tsp. lemon juice

½ tsp. or more superfood green (Vitamineral Green by Health Force, spirulina, chlorella or blue-green algae)

Sauté all ingredients, except superfood powder, in a pan for 5 minutes. Add superfood powder when finished cooking and mix well.

I love adding a superfood to many meals. It provides so many extra dense nutrients. Superfoods are great to travel with and to help you stay strong and vital. Spirulina, for instance, is very high in protein, chlorophyll, and lots of minerals and vitamins. A little bit goes a long way.

BLENDED SOUP

Serves: 2

2-½ c. cauliflower

2-½ c. water

½ tsp. sea salt

2 tbsp. olive oil

1/3 tsp. turmeric

2 c. kelp noodles

Steam cauliflower. Use ½ cup of the 2½ cups of steaming water and add to Vitamix with all of the other ingredients except the kelp noodles. Blend. Cut kelp noodles with scissors and put in a large bowl. Pour hot soup over noodles and mix. Let it sit for a few minutes to soften the noodles.

Kelp noodles are a great option if you like to eat noodles and do not do well with gluten or grains. They provide the consistency of a noodle, and are fun to eat.

Turmeric is great for the skin. It is anti-inflammatory, anti-oxidant, anti-cancer, and is a gentle liver cleanser. It is high in B6, riboflavin, iron, vitamin C, zinc, calcium, magnesium, and much more.

VEGGIES AND PROTEIN FOR CLEAR SKIN

Serves: 2

3 c. sautéed veggies (whatever suits your fancy, such as red cabbage, green cabbage, green peas, kale, broccoli, cauliflower, carrots, and Brussels sprouts)

1 piece protein of choice (again, whatever suits your fancy, such as wild-caught fish, wild-caught shrimp, or certain sustainably-raised fish or shrimp, 100% grass-fed meats, or pasture-raised chicken)

3 tsp. coconut oil

1 tsp. sea salt

1 tsp. vinegar of choice or lemon

Fresh herbs (as much as you like)

Sauté veggies on medium heat in 2 tsp. coconut oil for a few minutes or until it is the consistency you like. Some combinations of veggies will require a different amount of oil. Some will require different lengths of time cooking. Broccoli, Brussels sprouts, or cauliflower will take longer than kale and peas. I love combining a few veggies together.

In a separate pan, sauté protein in 1 tsp. coconut oil, lemon, and sea salt. Add to veggies.

This is a basic staple of mine. It balances the blood sugar and provides much nutrition, including great fats and vitamins and minerals.

SIMPLE DRINKS

SIMPLE LEMONADE FOR CLEAR SKIN
Serves: 1 or 2
1 liter filtered or spring water
½ c. lemon juice

This lemon water is a great way to start the day and to sip anytime. It will motivate you to drink more water because it is so yummy and invigorating.

JUICY JUICE
Serves: 3
1 bunch kale
2 peeled lemons
1 c. mint leaves
3 c. water

In a high-powered blender, blend all of the ingredients. Strain, using a nut milk bag.

Fresh juice is hydrating and refreshing, and it feeds your body many vital nutrients. This particular juice has a strong lemon flavor. Not only does it taste delicious, but it also has great benefits for your health. It awakens your cells and is high in Vitamin C, invigorating your immune system and skin. It gently cleanses the liver and has a great sour flavor.

HEMP MILK
Serves: 4
½ cup organic hemp seed
4 tsp. xylitol
1½ c. water
⅛ tsp. sea salt
1 vanilla bean

Take out all of the vanilla powder from the vanilla bean pod with a spoon. Blend all ingredients in Vitamix; no need to strain.

This can be added to tea or cereal; you can add cacao, or just drink it plain. Hemp milk is a super alternative to cow's milk or even rice milk. For a lot of people, drinking dairy is not beneficial, so a good option is such protein-rich alternatives as hemp milk.

HEALTHY SWEET TREATS

BANANA PUDDING
Serves: 2
2 bananas
½ avocado
1/3 tsp. ground cinnamon

Put all ingredients in a Vitamix and blend until smooth.

You can add cacao nibs on top, or any other fruit or nuts you desire. I love blueberries and strawberries.

This is a great treat with the exact consistency of pudding. It is soft and digestible, and is quick and easy to make. Cinnamon helps with blood-sugar balancing, so it is perfect to add to a dessert with a high glycemic fruit, such as banana. I love this when I want something delicious, sweet, and comforting. It has a very soothing quality and can be eaten when you are having a stomach challenge or not feeling great.

CHOCOLATE COOKIE DOUGH FOR CLEAR SKIN
Serves: 2
2 tbsp. sprouted almond butter
2 tbsp. organic tahini
2 tbsp. cacao nibs
2 tbsp. xylitol
¼ tsp. sea salt

Put all of the ingredients in a small bowl and mix together with a spoon. Form into small balls and eat right away. For a cold treat, store in fridge or freezer.

Sweet flavors are nourishing to our hearts. Eating something so rich in taste brings joy. I love that this is super delicious, simple, and also very nutritious.

Growing up, I remember noticing that I would get pimples when I ate chocolate and lots of sugar. Looking back, I believe it had to do with the quality of the chocolate. Eating conventional candy bars with cooked chocolate and high sugar content was the combination, I believe, that aggravated my skin. I still eat chocolate, but I choose raw cacao with low glycemic sweetener. This makes a big difference for me, and I rarely get any pimples. I created a dough-like treat that tastes amazing, is good for me, and is simple to make.

These recipes are a good resource for great tasting and very nutritious meals and treats. They use simple ingredients that go down smoothly and easily.

RECOMMENDED PRODUCTS

Here is a list of products and brands that I recommend. They are brands that I suggest regularly for the supplements that I've mentioned in this book. After years of working with many different products, I can say these are my favorite lines due to their excellent quality and efficacy.

HIGH QUALITY OILS:
Coconut Oil:
Brands: Sun Star Organics (online), Nutiva, Artisana

Fish Oil Supplement:
Brands: Liquid and Capsule: Pharmax, Nordic Naturals
Capsule: Renew Life

Krill Oil:
Brands: Capsule: Nature's Way, Dr. Mercola

Grass-fed Butter:
Brand: Organic Valley

Cacao Butter:
Brands: Navitas Naturals, Longevity Warehouse (online)

Olive Oil:
Brands: Olea Estates Organic Extra Virgin Olive Oil (online or farmers market in Boulder, Co), Bariani Olive Oil (online, some specialty stores)

Hemp Oil:
Brand: Nutiva

Fermented Cod Liver Oil:
Brand: Capsule or Liquid: Green Pasture

Evening Primrose Oil:
Brand: Capsule: Barleans

DIGESTIVE PRODUCTS:
Digestive Enzymes:
Brands: Capsule: Renew Life, Enzymedica, Doctor's Best

Probiotics:
Brands: Capsule: Renew Life, Mega Foods, Dr Ohira, Pharmax

L-glutamine:
Brand: Powder: Now

Chia Seeds:
Brands: Nutiva, Garden of Life

Herbs for Candida: Pau d'arco, Oregon Grape Root:
Brands: Tincture: Herb Pharm, Gaia

STRESS REMEDY PRODUCTS:
Flower Essences:
Brands: Liquid: Bach, FES

Rescue Remedy:
Brand: Liquid: Bach

B Vitamins:
Brands: Tablet: Mega Foods
Capsule: Pure Encapsulation, Premier Research Labs (online, pharmacies, wellness clinics or healthcare practitioners)

Reishi:
Brands: Capsule: Dragon Herbs, Host Defense, Mushroom Science

Tulsi (also called Holy Basil):
Brands: Bulk Herb: Mountain Rose
Tea: Tea Bags: Organic India
Capsule: Organic India, Paradise Herbs

Oatstraw:
Brand: Bulk Herb: Mountain Rose

Ashwaganda Root:
Brands: Bulk herb: Mountain Rose
Tincture: Herb Pharm
Capsule: Organic India, Gaia, Paradise Herbs

Motherwort:
Brands: Bulk Herb: Mountain Rose
Tincture: Herb Pharm

Passionflower:
Brands: Bulk Herb: Mountain Rose
Tincture: Herb Pharm
Capsule: Paradise Herbs, Gaia

L- Theanine:
Brands: Capsule: Paradise Herbs, Dragon Herbs (the product is called 'Tao in a Bottle')

IMMUNITY PRODUCTS:
Medicinal Mushrooms:
Brands: Capsule: Dragon Herbs, Host Defense, Mushroom Science

Cordyceps:
Brands: Capsule: Host Defense, Mushroom Science, Dragon Herbs

Turmeric:
Brands: Tincture: Herb Pharm
Capsule: New Chapter
Powder: Mega Foods

Olive Leaf:
Brands: Capsule: Premier Research Labs (online and refer above), Gaia
Tincture: Gaia

Nettles:
Brands: Capsule: Eclectic, Gaia
Tincture: Gaia, Herb Pharm

Astragalus Root:
Brands: Capsule: Paradise Herbs
Tincture: Herb Pharm, Gaia

Vitamin D:
Brands: Liquid: Premier Research Labs (online and refer above), Rx Vitamins
Capsule: Jarrow

Vitamin C:
Brands: Powder: HealthForce Nutritionals
Tablet and Powder: Mega Foods

Zinc:
Brands: Tablet: Mega Food
Liquid: Trace Minerals, Mineral Life (online)

Colostrum:
Brand: Capsule: Pure Encapsulations

Chinese Mountain Ant:
Brand: Liquid and Capsule: Dragon Herbs

LIVER PRODUCTS:
Dandelion, Red clover, Burdock root, Oregon grape root, Milk thistle seed:
Brands: Herbs in bulk: Mountain Rose
Tincture: Herb Pharm, Gaia

OTHER PRODUCTS:
Nascent Iodine:
Brand: Liquid: LL's Magnetic Clay Inc.

Essential Oils:
Brands: Young Living, doTerra (online), Living Libations (online and some stores), Wyndmere

MSM:
Brands: Powder: Jarrow, Omica (online)

SUPERFOODS:
Blue-green algae:
Brand: Powder: HealthForce Nutritionals

Lacuma:
Brand: Powder: Navitas Naturals

Camu Camu:
Brand: Powder: Navitas Naturals

Cacao Powder or Nibs:
Brands: Navitas Naturals, Longevity Warehouse (online)

Seaweed:
Brands: Marine Coast Sea Veggie, Emerald Cove

Chlorella:
Brands: Powder or Tablet: HealthForce Nutritionals
Tablets: Sunfood Superfoods

Spirulina:
Brands: Powder or Tablets: HealthForce Nutritionals
Powder: Longevity Warehouse (online)

Hemp Seed:
Brands: Manitoba Harvest, Nutiva

OTHER FOODS:
Irish Moss:
Brand: Sun Star Organics (online)

Stevia:
Brand: Liquid or Powder: Omica

Honey:
Brands: Omica, Longevity Warehouse (online)

Kelp Noodles:
Brand: Sea Tangle

Xylitol (Birch):
Brands: Ultimate Life, Morning Pep

Coconut Sugar:
Brand: Coconut Secrets

Coconut Flour:
Brands: Coconut Secret, Edwards and Sons, Nutiva

Pea Chips:
Brand: Goldmine

Crackers:
Brand: Jilz

TOPICAL OPTIONS:
Burdock Root, Oregon Grape Root:
Brand: Bulk herb: Mountain Rose

Product name: Psorzema Cream
Brand: Derma E

REFERENCES

1. *The Vortex: Where the Law of Attraction Assembles All Cooperative Relationships*, Esther and Jerry Hicks, Hay House, 2009

2. *Rawsome*, Brigitte Mars, Basic Health Publications, 2004

3. *The Desktop Guide to Herbal Medicine*, Brigitte Mars, Basic Health Publications, 2007

4. *The Home Reference to Holistic Health and Healing: Easy-To-Use Natural Remedies, Herb, Flower Essences, Essential Oils, Supplements, and Therapeutic Practices for Health, Happiness, and Well-Being, Brigitte Mars*, Fair Winds Press, 2014

5. *You Can Heal Your Life*, Louise Hay, Hay House, 1999

6. *Loving What Is: Four Questions That Can Change Your Life*, Byron Katie, Crown Publishing Group, 2002

7. "How To Stop Attacking Yourself: 9 Steps To Heal Autoimmune Disease.", Dr. Mark Hyman, an article, updated 2013

8. *Taming Your Gremlin*, Rick Carson, HarperCollins Publisher, 2009

9. *Practical Paleo*, Diane Sanfilippo, Victory Belt Publishing Inc, 2012

10. *Eating In The Light Of The Moon: How Women Can Transform Their Relationship With Food Through Myths, Metaphors, and Storytelling*, Dr. Anita Johnston, Gurze Books, 2000

11. Guttate Psoriasis Often Linked to Strep Throat, Guttate Mostly Affects Young People, Rosalyn Carson-DeWitt, an article, About.com Psoriasis, 2008

12. Plaque Psoriasis, National Psoriasis Foundation, psoriasis.org, an article

13. Guttate Psoriasis, reviewed by Deborah Jaliman MD, an article, Web MD, Psoriasis Health Center, 2013

14. Natural Immune Modulators May Provide a Key to Beating Immune Disorders, Toni Isaacs, an article, Natural News, 2011

15. Balancing Your Body's pH Levels, Liz Barrington, an article, Natural Body Healing Restoring Health and Harmony to Your Body

16. 9 Ways To Eliminate Sugar Cravings, Jacqueline Sylvestri Banks, an article, Fox News, 2013

17. *Eating for Beauty,* David Wolfe, North Atlantic Books, 2002

18. *The Sunfood Diet Success System,* David Wolfe, North Atlantic Books, 1999

19. Psoriasis as an Autoimmune Disorder, Rosalyn Carson-DeWitt, an article, About.com Psoriasis, 2009 (updated)

20. *The Flowering of Human Consciousness,* Eckhart Tolle, Audio CD, DVD, Sounds True, 2004

21. *Living the Liberated Life and Dealing With the Pain Body,* Eckhart Tolle, Audio CD, Sounds True, 2001

22. *The Power of Now: A Guide to Spiritual Enlightenment,* Eckhart Tolle, Namaste Publishing, 1997

23. *A New Earth,* Eckhart Tolle, Plume, 2005

24. *The Realization of Being*, Eckhart Tolle, Audio CD, Sounds True, 2001

25. What is Nascent Iodine?, Dr. Edward Group, Global Healing Center, 2012, last updated 2015

26. Autoimmune Disorders and Digestive Health, Dr. Ionela Hubbard, an article, Integrative Functional Medicine and Acupuncture Center

27. *Amazing Grace*, David Wolfe and Nick Good, North Atlantic books, 2008

28. *JingSlingets' Food With Benefits*, Joy Coelho and Jay Denman, WaterStone Media, 2015

29. Sprouting Nuts and Seed, Diana Herrington, an article, www.care2.com, 2011

30. *The Secret*, Rhonda Byrne, Atria Books, Beyond Words Publishing, 2006

Author's Bio

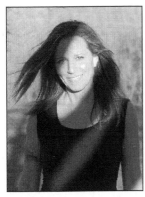

MARJY BERKMAN HAS A STRONG passion for helping others live in vibrant health. She is an author, Certified Clinical Herbalist, Certified Nutritionist, Raw Food Chef, and Licensed Massage Therapist. Marjy's consultations have for fifteen years helped people with skin challenges and other health issues find peace and ease with their situation. She facilitates her clients in healing their skin by playing with ways to optimize their nutrition and supporting them in finding the way to inner and outer alignment.

Marjy offers both nutritional and spiritual consulting. She can be reached at mjberkman@yahoo.com or http://www.SkinSoulutions.com

Made in the USA
Lexington, KY
22 September 2018